Get Healthy with Color

~Health Logs and Coloring Art~

Written and Illustrated by

SANDRA KEEN

ISBN: 0-9978690-2-X
ISBN-13: 978-0-9978690-2-6

Disclaimer

Anyone beginning a new exercise regimen or diet plan should first seek medical advice from their doctor or medical practitioner. Similarly, prior to a new exercise regimen, blood pressure readings should also be reviewed with medical practitioners or doctors so that the best plan of care can be prescribed for you. Please also note that your doctor or medical practitioner may suggest specific exercises as well as blood pressure measurement routines that are best for you. Adherence to such medical plans of care are crucial to effective health management and prevention. This log book is intended only to help keep track of health initiatives. Extra space is also available on this log for additional health initiatives that may be prescribed.

Notice

Contact

Inquiries regarding this or other publications by Keen Inspirational Media, Sandra Keen, Jessie Keen, Michael Keen, or Milton Keen should be directed to Sandra@keeninspirationalmedia.com.

DEDICATION

Dedicated to A Healthier and Happier You!

COLORING WITH PURPOSE

There are many apps that help to track daily exercise regimens. So many varieties, in fact, by so many providers. For those who love to color and prefer a more tactile journaling experience, this journal is for you! It is intended to add another layer of joy on the journey to better health. Add to it, use the margins, color, and be creative. This is YOUR journal. Enjoy your journey to a healthier and happier you!

COMPLETING YOUR JOURNAL
ACHIEVING YOUR GOALS

A few things to keep in mind when completing your journal. Many people find that taking time to color is a relaxing stress reliever. It is equally important to dedicate enough time to move. For this reason, some daily drawings are more simple than others. The more complicated drawings are spread throughout this journal to allow more time to revisit them after taking time for a walk or to fit in a workout. Please enjoy your journal, your exercise, and your better health. Enjoy a routine that works for you.

Remember to consult your physician before beginning a new exercise regimen.

Day / Date : _____

Meal	Details	Calories
Breakfast		
Snack		
Lunch		
Snack		
Dinner		

Exercise	Time	Wt.	Sets/Reps
			/
			/
			/
			/
			/
			/
			/
			/
			/
			/
			/
			/

Today's Results :

Blood Pressure /Time/Pulse :

/   __:__   _____
/   __:__   _____

Today's Weight :

Total Calories :

Water Intake :

Current Medications / Supplements :

What Inspired Me Today? (Ex: A Person, Goal Achieved, A Quote, or Misc.) :

My Progress Notes :

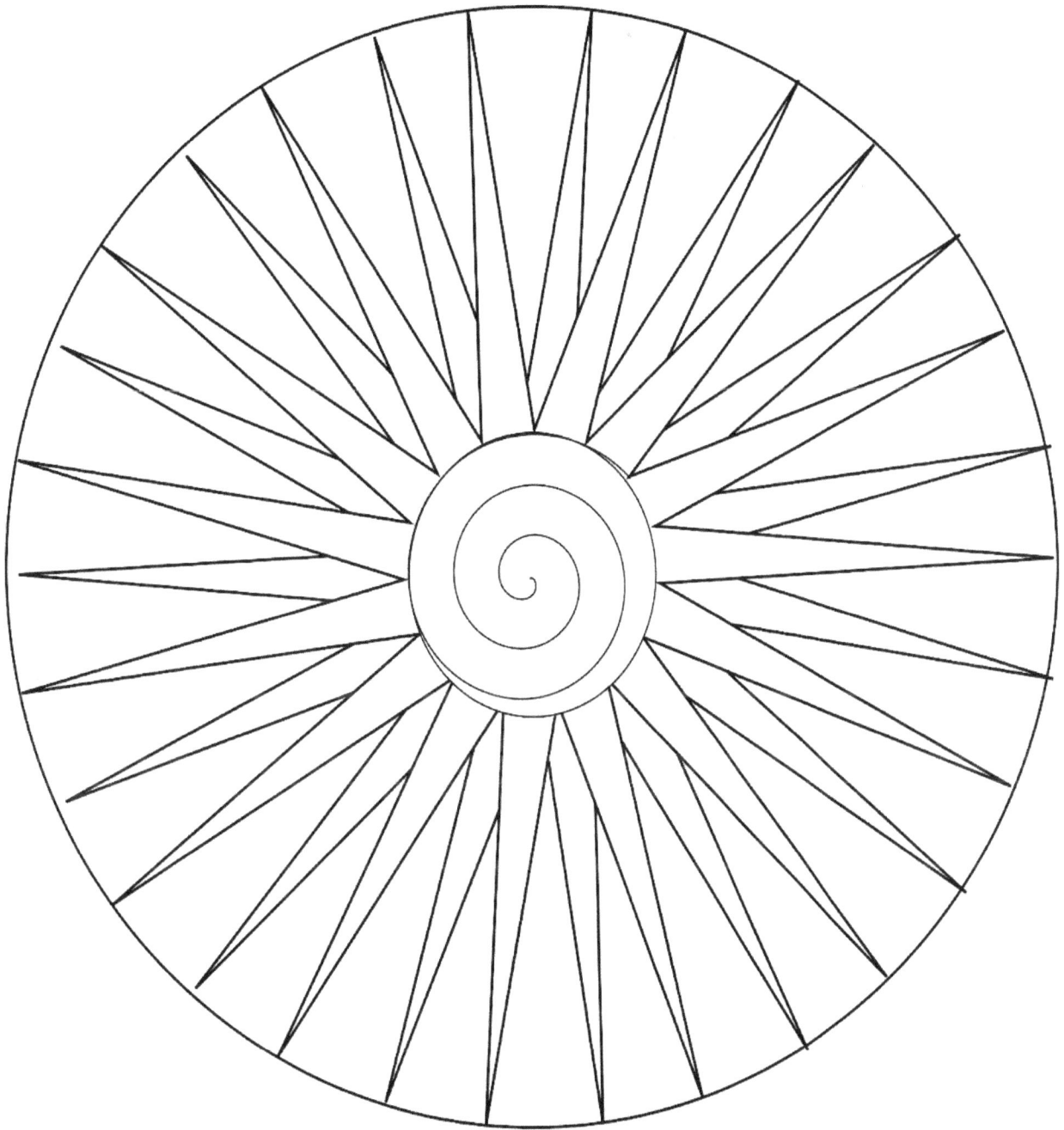

Day / Date : _____

Meal	Details	Calories
Breakfast		
Snack		
Lunch		
Snack		
Dinner		

Exercise	Time	Wt.	Sets/Reps
			/
			/
			/
			/
			/
			/
			/
			/
			/
			/
			/
			/

Today's Results :

Blood Pressure /Time/Pulse :

/   __:__   _____

/   __:__   _____

Today's Weight :

Total Calories :

Water Intake :

Current Medications / Supplements :

What Inspired Me Today? (Ex: A Person, Goal Achieved, A Quote, or Misc.) :

My Progress Notes :

My Progress Reflections
& General Inspirations

_____

_____

_____

_____

_____

_____

_____

_____

_____

_____

_____

_____

_____

_____

_____

Day / Date : _____

Meal	Details	Calories		Exercise	Time	Wt.	Sets/Reps
Breakfast							/
Snack							/
Lunch							/
Snack							/
Dinner							/
							/
							/
							/
							/
							/
							/
							/
							/

Today's Results :

Blood Pressure / Time/Pulse :
/ ___:___ _____
/ ___:___ _____

Today's Weight :

Total Calories :

Water Intake :

Current Medications / Supplements :

What Inspired Me Today? (Ex: A Person, Goal Achieved, A Quote, or Misc.) :

My Progress Notes :

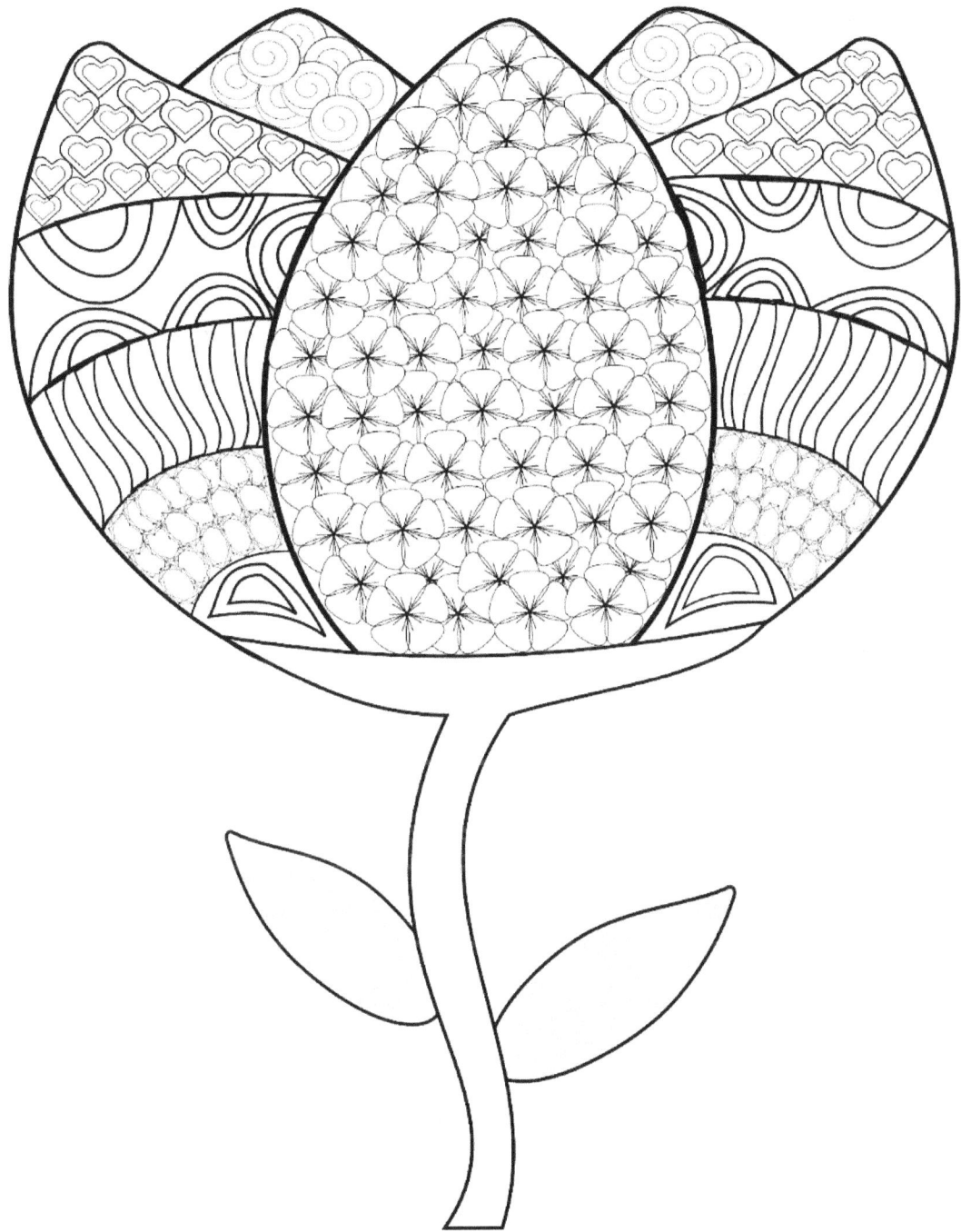

Day / Date : _____

Meal	Details	Calories
Breakfast		
Snack		
Lunch		
Snack		
Dinner		

Today's Results :

Blood Pressure /Time/Pulse : / __:__ _____ / __:__ _____	
Today's Weight :	
Total Calories :	
Water Intake :	
Current Medications / Supplements :	

Exercise	Time	Wt.	Sets/Reps
			/
			/
			/
			/
			/
			/
			/
			/
			/
			/
			/

What Inspired Me Today? (Ex: A Person, Goal Achieved, A Quote, or Misc.) :

My Progress Notes :

My Progress Reflections
& General Inspirations

_____

_____

_____

_____

_____

_____

_____

_____

_____

_____

_____

_____

_____

_____

_____

_____

Day / Date : _____

Meal	Details	Calories
Breakfast		
Snack		
Lunch		
Snack		
Dinner		

Exercise	Time	Wt.	Sets/Reps
			/
			/
			/
			/
			/
			/
			/
			/
			/
			/
			/
			/

Today's Results :

Blood Pressure /Time/Pulse :
/   __:__   _____
/   __:__   _____

Today's Weight :

Total Calories :

Water Intake :

Current Medications / Supplements :

What Inspired Me Today? (Ex: A Person, Goal Achieved, A Quote, or Misc.) :

My Progress Notes :

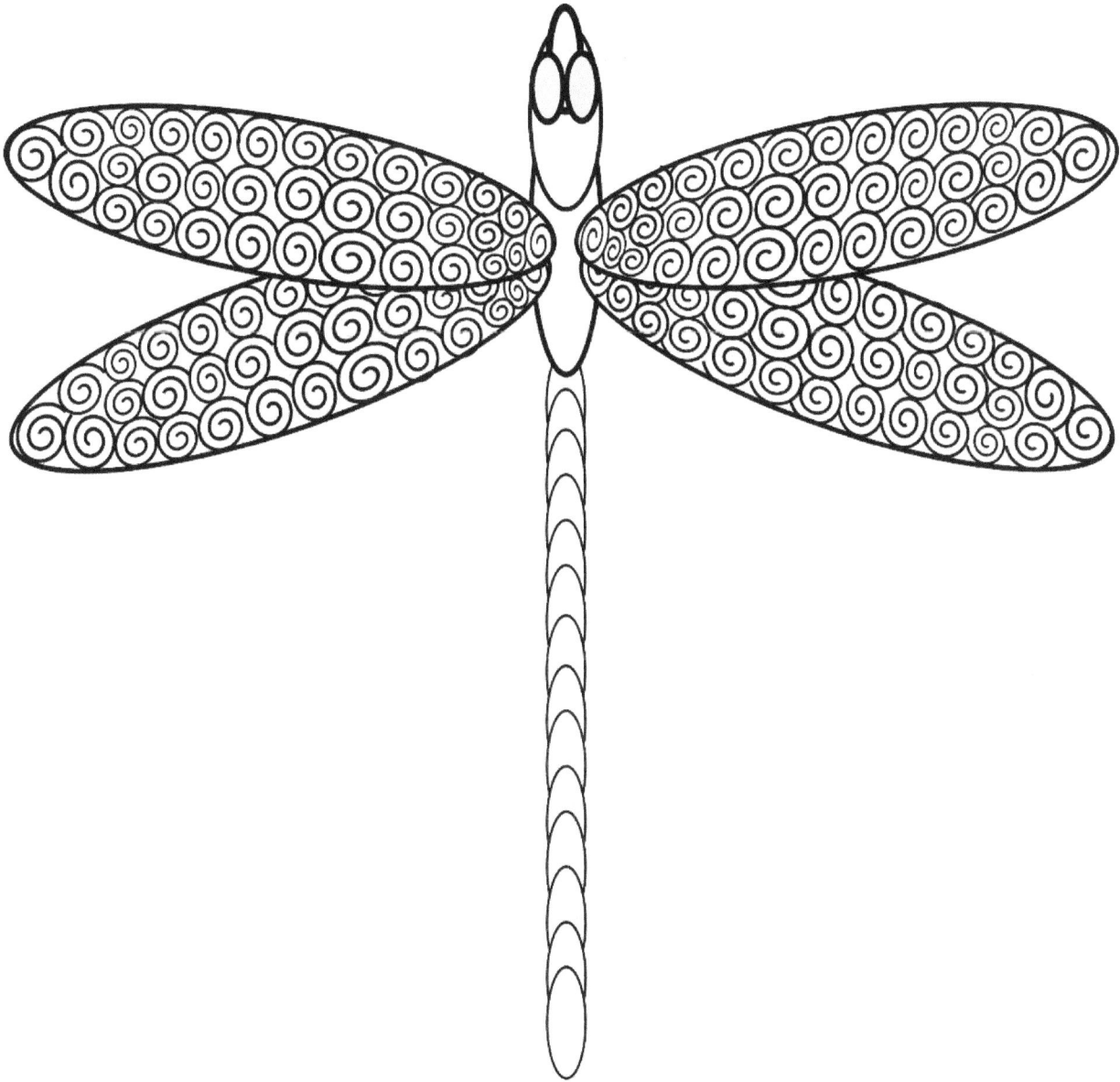

Day / Date : _____

Meal	Details	Calories
Breakfast		
Snack		
Lunch		
Snack		
Dinner		

Exercise	Time	Wt.	Sets/Reps
			/
			/
			/
			/
			/
			/
			/
			/
			/
			/
			/

Today's Results :

Blood Pressure /Time/Pulse :

    /   __:__   _____
    /   __:__   _____

Today's Weight :

Total Calories :

Water Intake :

Current Medications / Supplements :

What Inspired Me Today? (Ex: A Person, Goal Achieved, A Quote, or Misc.) :

My Progress Notes :

My Progress Reflections
& General Inspirations

_____

_____

_____

_____

_____

_____

_____

_____

_____

_____

_____

_____

_____

_____

_____

_____

_____

Day / Date : _____

Meal	Details	Calories
Breakfast		
Snack		
Lunch		
Snack		
Dinner		

Exercise	Time	Wt.	Sets/Reps
			/
			/
			/
			/
			/
			/
			/
			/
			/
			/
			/

Today's Results :

Blood Pressure /Time/Pulse :

    /   __:__   _____

    /   __:__   _____

Today's Weight :

Total Calories :

Water Intake :

Current Medications / Supplements :

What Inspired Me Today? (Ex: A Person, Goal Achieved, A Quote, or Misc.) :

My Progress Notes :

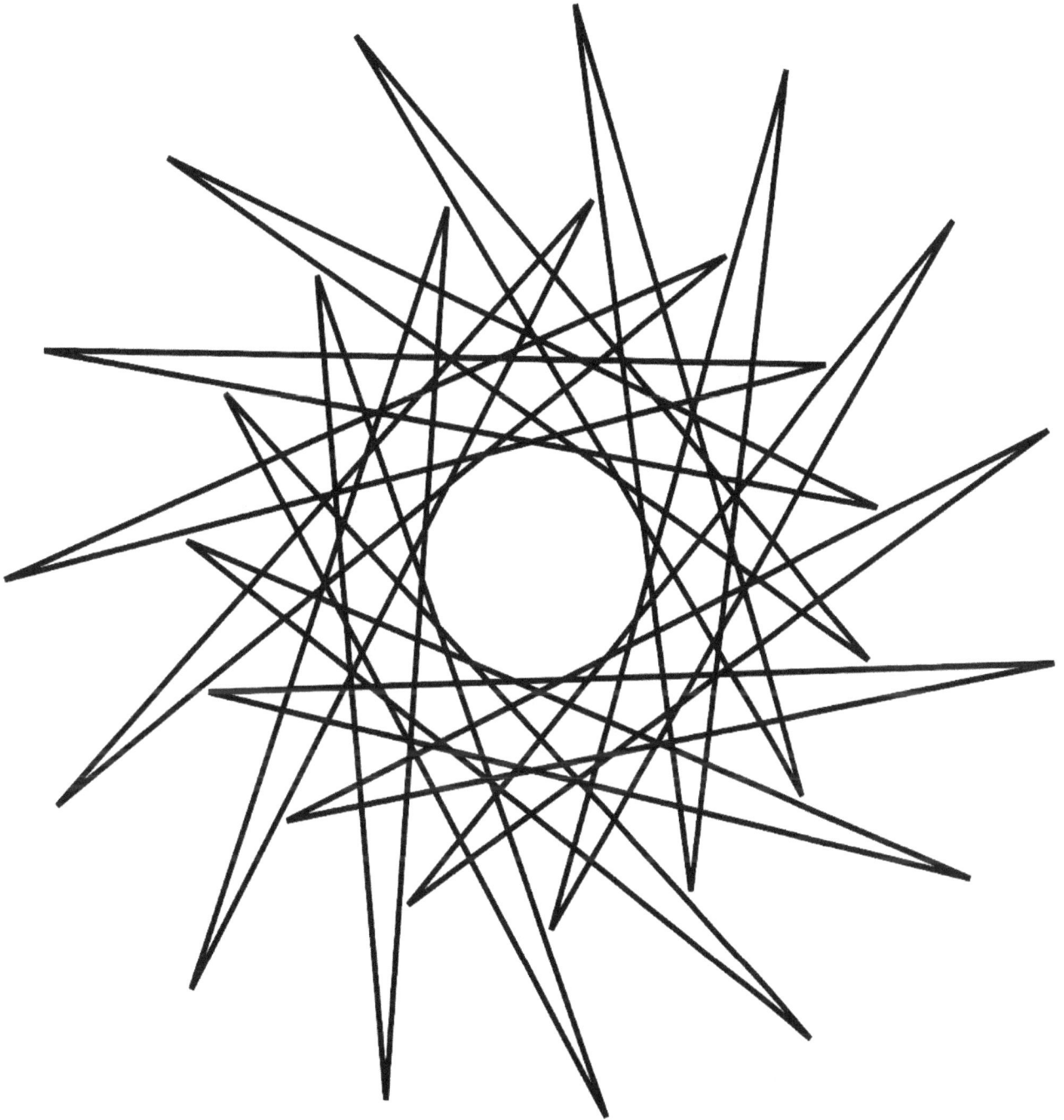

Day / Date : _____

Meal	Details	Calories
Breakfast		
Snack		
Lunch		
Snack		
Dinner		

Exercise	Time	Wt.	Sets/Reps
			/
			/
			/
			/
			/
			/
			/
			/
			/
			/
			/
			/

Today's Results :

Blood Pressure /Time/Pulse :

/   __:__   _____
/   __:__   _____

Today's Weight :

Total Calories :

Water Intake :

Current Medications / Supplements :

What Inspired Me Today? (Ex: A Person, Goal Achieved, A Quote, or Misc.) :

My Progress Notes :

My Progress Reflections
& General Inspirations

_____

_____

_____

_____

_____

_____

_____

_____

_____

_____

_____

_____

_____

_____

_____

Day / Date : _____

Meal	Details	Calories		Exercise	Time	Wt.	Sets/Reps
Breakfast							/
Snack							/
Lunch							/
Snack							/
Dinner							/
							/
							/
							/
							/

Today's Results :

Blood Pressure / Time / Pulse :

/ ___:___ _____
/ ___:___ _____

Today's Weight :

Total Calories :

Water Intake :

Current Medications / Supplements :

What Inspired Me Today? (Ex: A Person, Goal Achieved, A Quote, or Misc.) :

_____
_____
_____
_____

My Progress Notes :

_____
_____
_____
_____

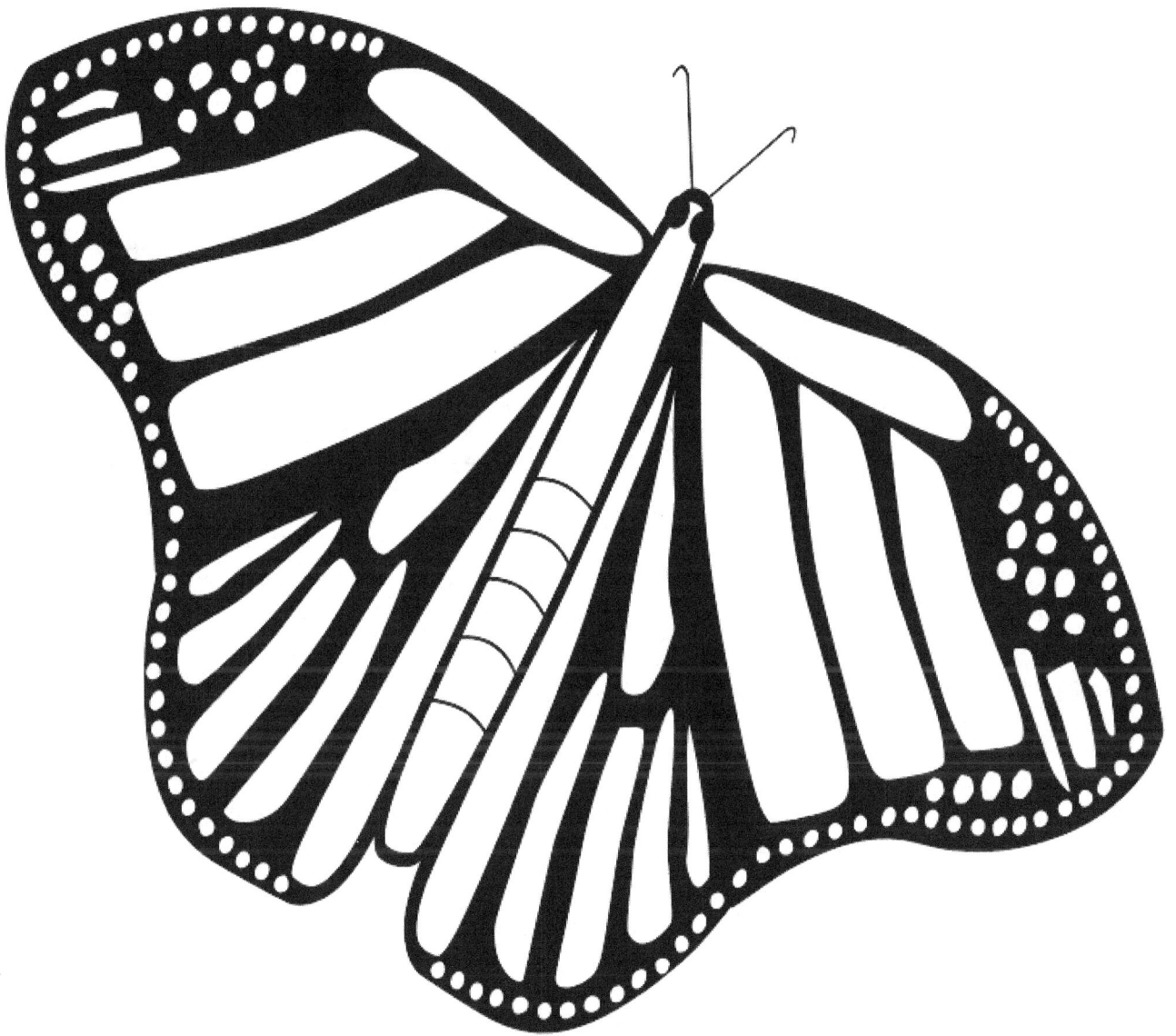

Day / Date : _____

Meal	Details	Calories
Breakfast		
Snack		
Lunch		
Snack		
Dinner		

Exercise	Time	Wt.	Sets/Reps
			/
			/
			/
			/
			/
			/
			/
			/
			/
			/
			/

Today's Results :

Blood Pressure / Time / Pulse :

/ ___:___ _____
/ ___:___ _____

Today's Weight :

Total Calories :

Water Intake :

Current Medications / Supplements :

What Inspired Me Today? (Ex: A Person, Goal Achieved, A Quote, or Misc.) :

My Progress Notes :

My Progress Reflections
& General Inspirations

_____

_____

_____

_____

_____

_____

_____

_____

_____

_____

_____

_____

_____

_____

_____

Day / Date : _____

Meal	Details	Calories		Exercise	Time	Wt.	Sets/Reps
Breakfast							
							/
Snack							/
Lunch							/
							/
Snack							/
Dinner							/
							/

Today's Results :		Exercise	Time	Wt.	Sets/Reps
Blood Pressure /Time/Pulse : / __:__ _____ / __:__ _____					/
					/
Today's Weight :					/
Total Calories :					/
Water Intake :					/
Current Medications / Supplements :					/

What Inspired Me Today? (Ex: A Person, Goal Achieved, A Quote, or Misc.) :

_____

_____

_____

_____

My Progress Notes :

_____

_____

_____

_____

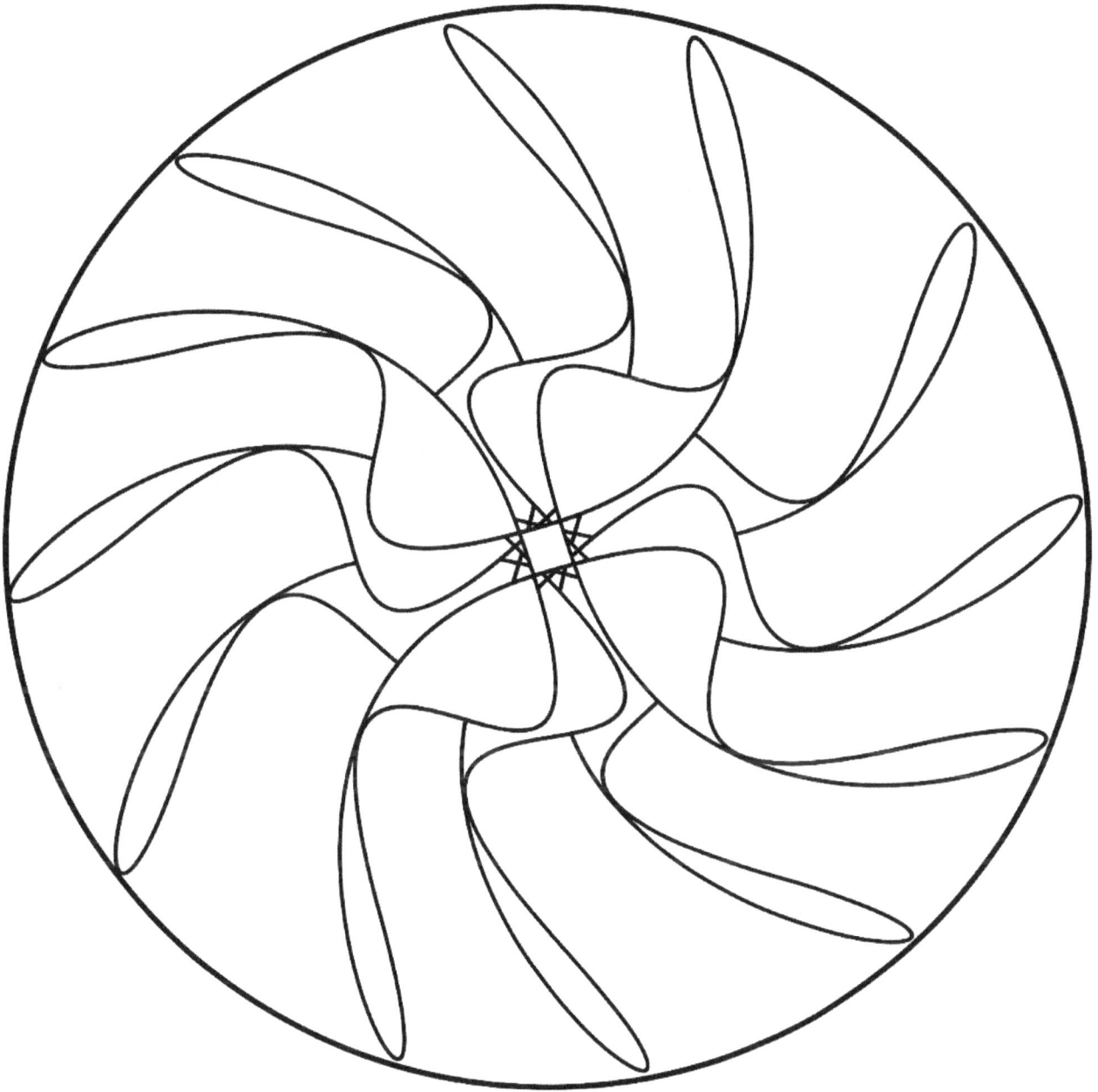

Day / Date : _____

Meal	Details	Calories
Breakfast		
Snack		
Lunch		
Snack		
Dinner		

Exercise	Time	Wt.	Sets/Reps
			/
			/
			/
			/
			/
			/
			/
			/
			/
			/
			/
			/

Today's Results :

Blood Pressure /Time/Pulse :

/ ___:___ _____

/ ___:___ _____

Today's Weight :

Total Calories :

Water Intake :

Current Medications / Supplements :

What Inspired Me Today? (Ex: A Person, Goal Achieved, A Quote, or Misc.) :

My Progress Notes :

My Progress Reflections
& General Inspirations

_____

_____

_____

_____

_____

_____

_____

_____

_____

_____

_____

_____

_____

_____

_____

_____

Day / Date : _____

Meal	Details	Calories
Breakfast		
Snack		
Lunch		
Snack		
Dinner		

Exercise	Time	Wt.	Sets/Reps
			/
			/
			/
			/
			/
			/
			/
			/
			/
			/
			/
			/

Today's Results :

Blood Pressure /Time/Pulse :

/ ___:___ _____
/ ___:___ _____

Today's Weight :

Total Calories :

Water Intake :

Current Medications / Supplements :

What Inspired Me Today? (Ex: A Person, Goal Achieved, A Quote, or Misc.) :

_____
_____
_____
_____

My Progress Notes :

_____
_____
_____
_____

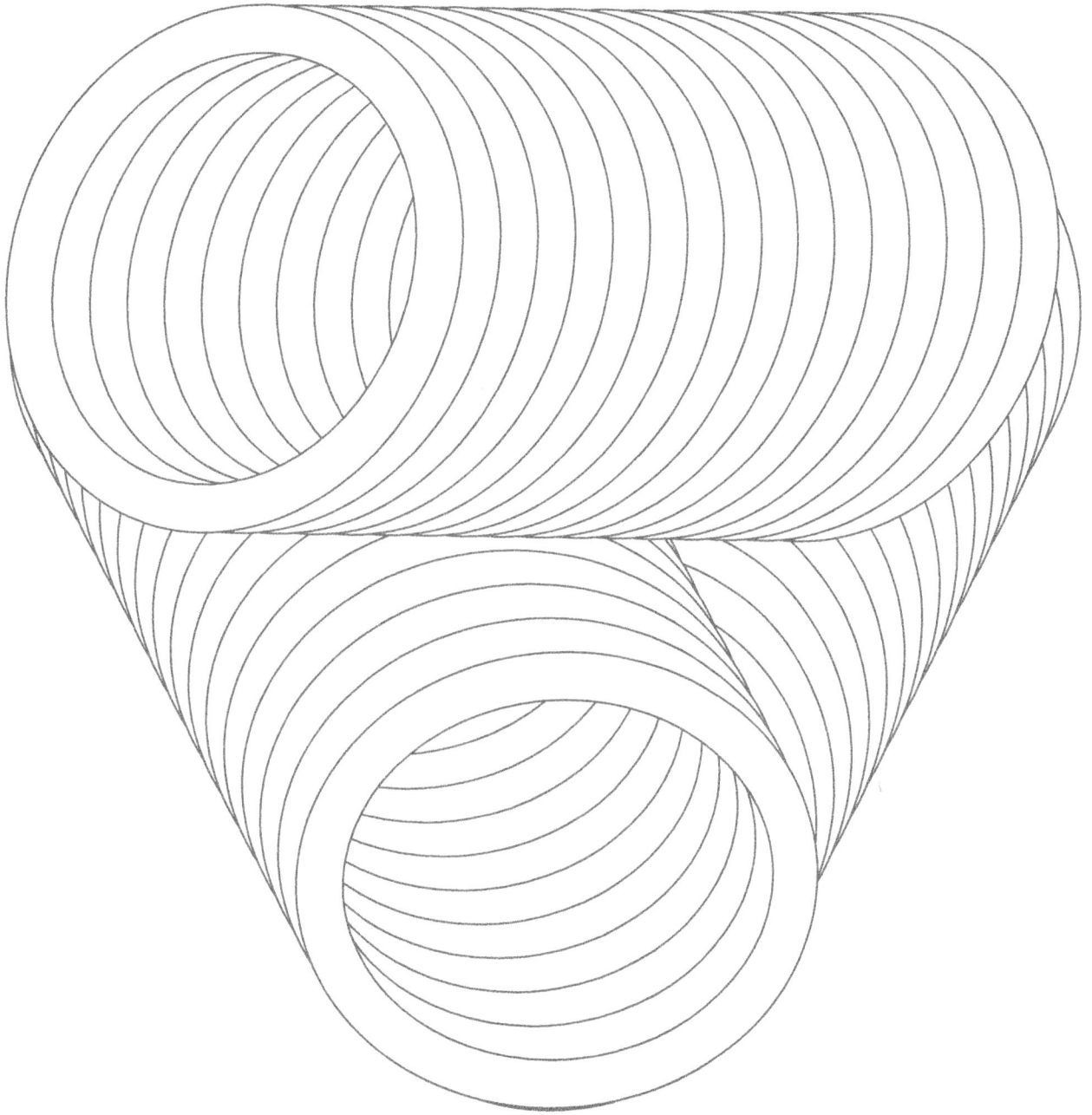

Day / Date : _____

Meal	Details	Calories
Breakfast		
Snack		
Lunch		
Snack		
Dinner		

Exercise	Time	Wt.	Sets/Reps
			/
			/
			/
			/
			/
			/
			/
			/
			/
			/
			/
			/

Today's Results :

Blood Pressure /Time/Pulse :

/ ___:___ _____
/ ___:___ _____

Today's Weight :

Total Calories :

Water Intake :

Current Medications / Supplements :

What Inspired Me Today? (Ex: A Person, Goal Achieved, A Quote, or Misc.) :

My Progress Notes :

My Progress Reflections
& General Inspirations

_____

_____

_____

_____

_____

_____

_____

_____

_____

_____

_____

_____

_____

_____

_____

_____

Day / Date : _____

Meal	Details	Calories
Breakfast		
Snack		
Lunch		
Snack		
Dinner		

Exercise	Time	Wt.	Sets/Reps
			/
			/
			/
			/
			/
			/
			/
			/
			/
			/
			/

Today's Results :

Blood Pressure / Time / Pulse :

/   __:__   _____

/   __:__   _____

Today's Weight :

Total Calories :

Water Intake :

Current Medications / Supplements :

What Inspired Me Today? (Ex: A Person, Goal Achieved, A Quote, or Misc.) :

My Progress Notes :

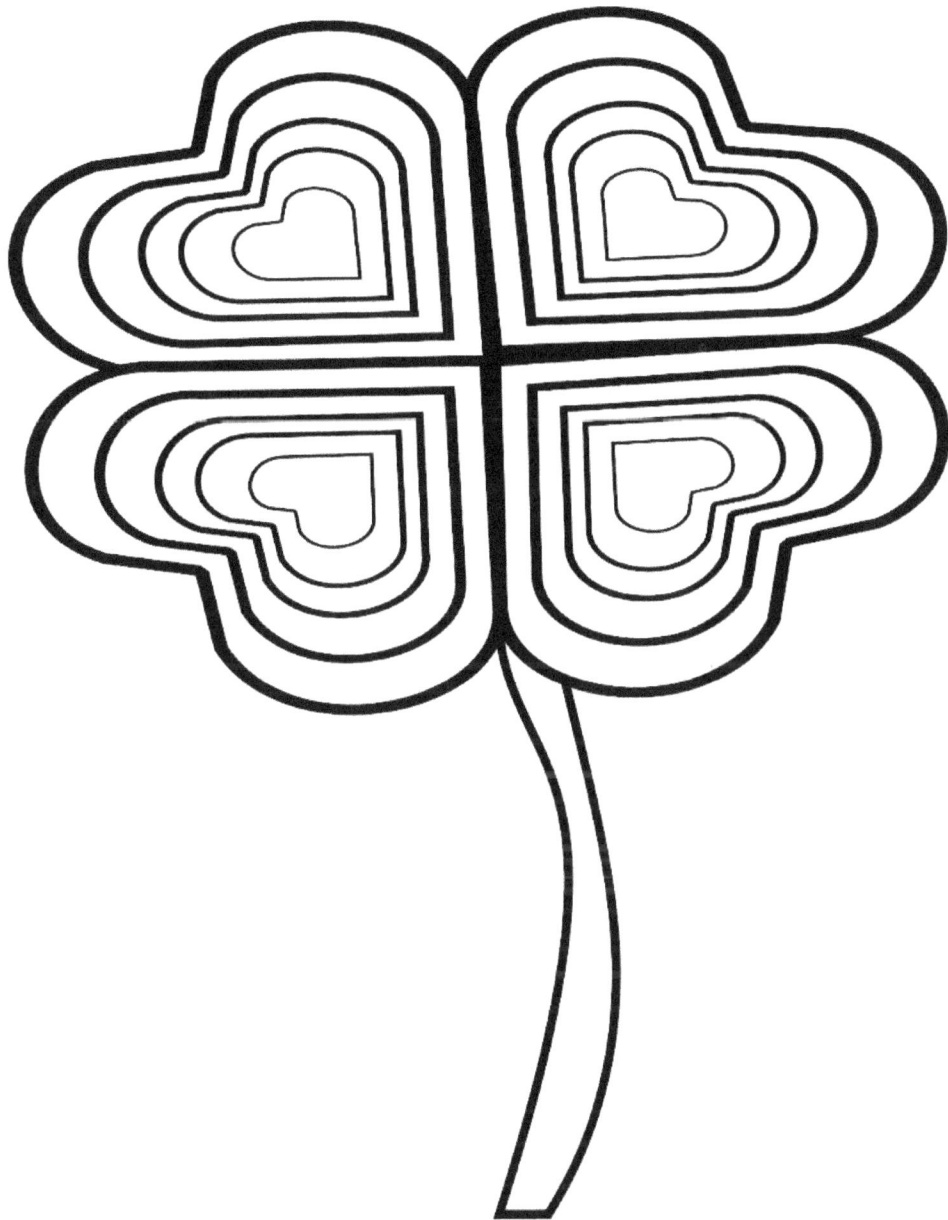

Day / Date : _____

Meal	Details	Calories
Breakfast		
Snack		
Lunch		
Snack		
Dinner		

Exercise	Time	Wt.	Sets/Reps
			/
			/
			/
			/
			/
			/
			/
			/
			/
			/
			/

Today's Results :

Blood Pressure / Time / Pulse :

/   __:__   _____

/   __:__   _____

Today's Weight :

Total Calories :

Water Intake :

Current Medications / Supplements :

What Inspired Me Today? (Ex: A Person, Goal Achieved, A Quote, or Misc.) :

My Progress Notes :

My Progress Reflections
& General Inspirations

_____

_____

_____

_____

_____

_____

_____

_____

_____

_____

_____

_____

_____

_____

_____

_____

Day / Date : _____

Meal	Details	Calories
Breakfast		
Snack		
Lunch		
Snack		
Dinner		

Exercise	Time	Wt.	Sets/Reps
			/
			/
			/
			/
			/
			/
			/
			/
			/
			/
			/
			/

Today's Results :

Blood Pressure /Time/Pulse :
  / _____   __:__   _____
  / _____   __:__   _____

Today's Weight :

Total Calories :

Water Intake :

Current Medications / Supplements :

What Inspired Me Today? (Ex: A Person, Goal Achieved, A Quote, or Misc.) :

My Progress Notes :

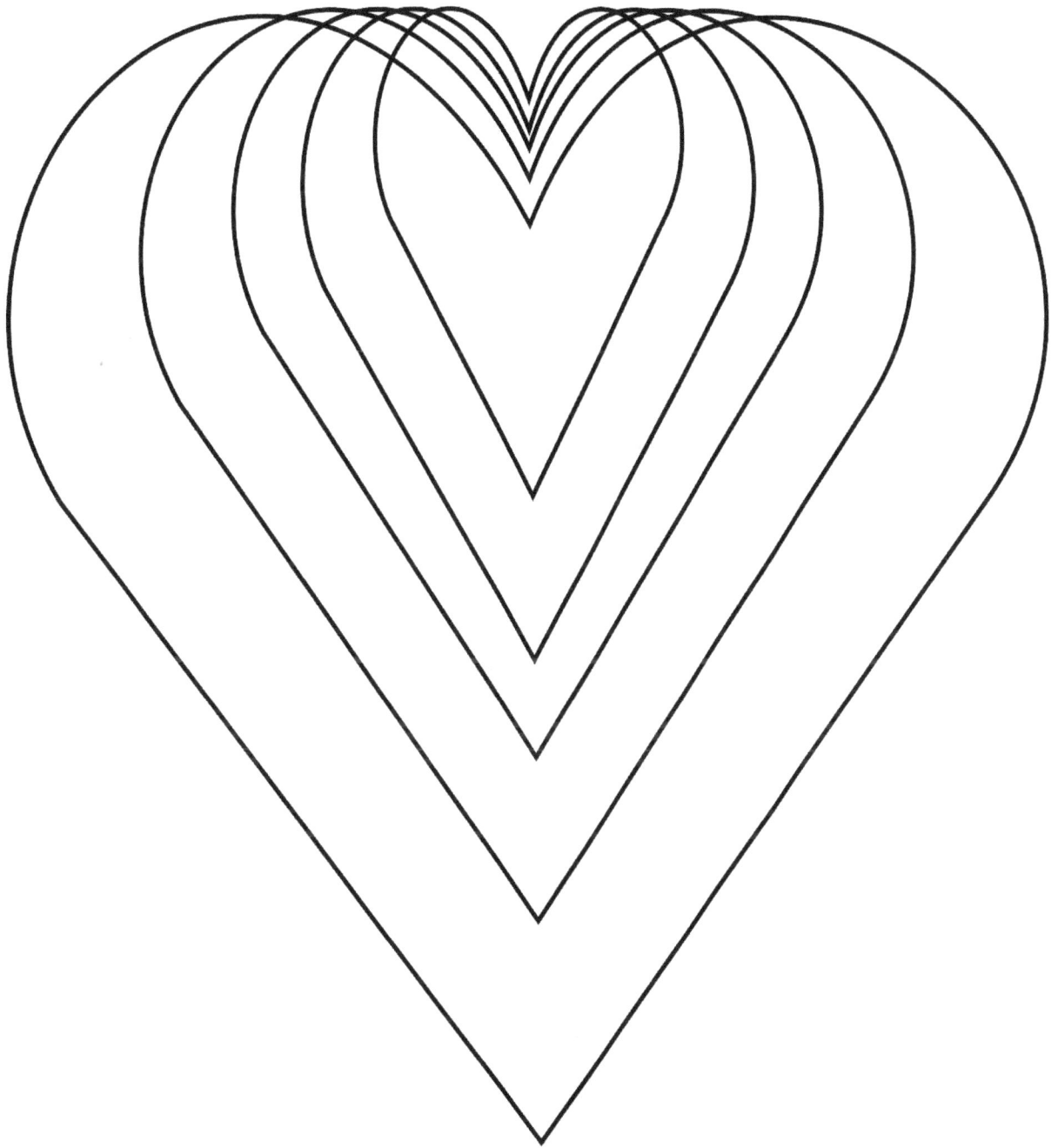

Day / Date : _____

Meal	Details	Calories
Breakfast		
Snack		
Lunch		
Snack		
Dinner		

Exercise	Time	Wt.	Sets/Reps
			/
			/
			/
			/
			/
			/
			/
			/
			/
			/
			/
			/

Today's Results :

Blood Pressure / Time / Pulse :

/ __:__ _____

/ __:__ _____

Today's Weight :

Total Calories :

Water Intake :

Current Medications / Supplements :

What Inspired Me Today? (Ex: A Person, Goal Achieved, A Quote, or Misc.) :

My Progress Notes :

My Progress Reflections & General Inspirations

_____

_____

_____

_____

_____

_____

_____

_____

_____

_____

_____

_____

_____

_____

_____

_____

Day / Date : _____

Meal	Details	Calories
Breakfast		
Snack		
Lunch		
Snack		
Dinner		

Exercise	Time	Wt.	Sets/Reps
			/
			/
			/
			/
			/
			/
			/
			/
			/
			/
			/
			/

Today's Results :

Blood Pressure /Time/Pulse :

/   __:__   _____

/   __:__   _____

Today's Weight :

Total Calories :

Water Intake :

Current Medications / Supplements :

What Inspired Me Today? (Ex: A Person, Goal Achieved, A Quote, or Misc.) :

My Progress Notes :

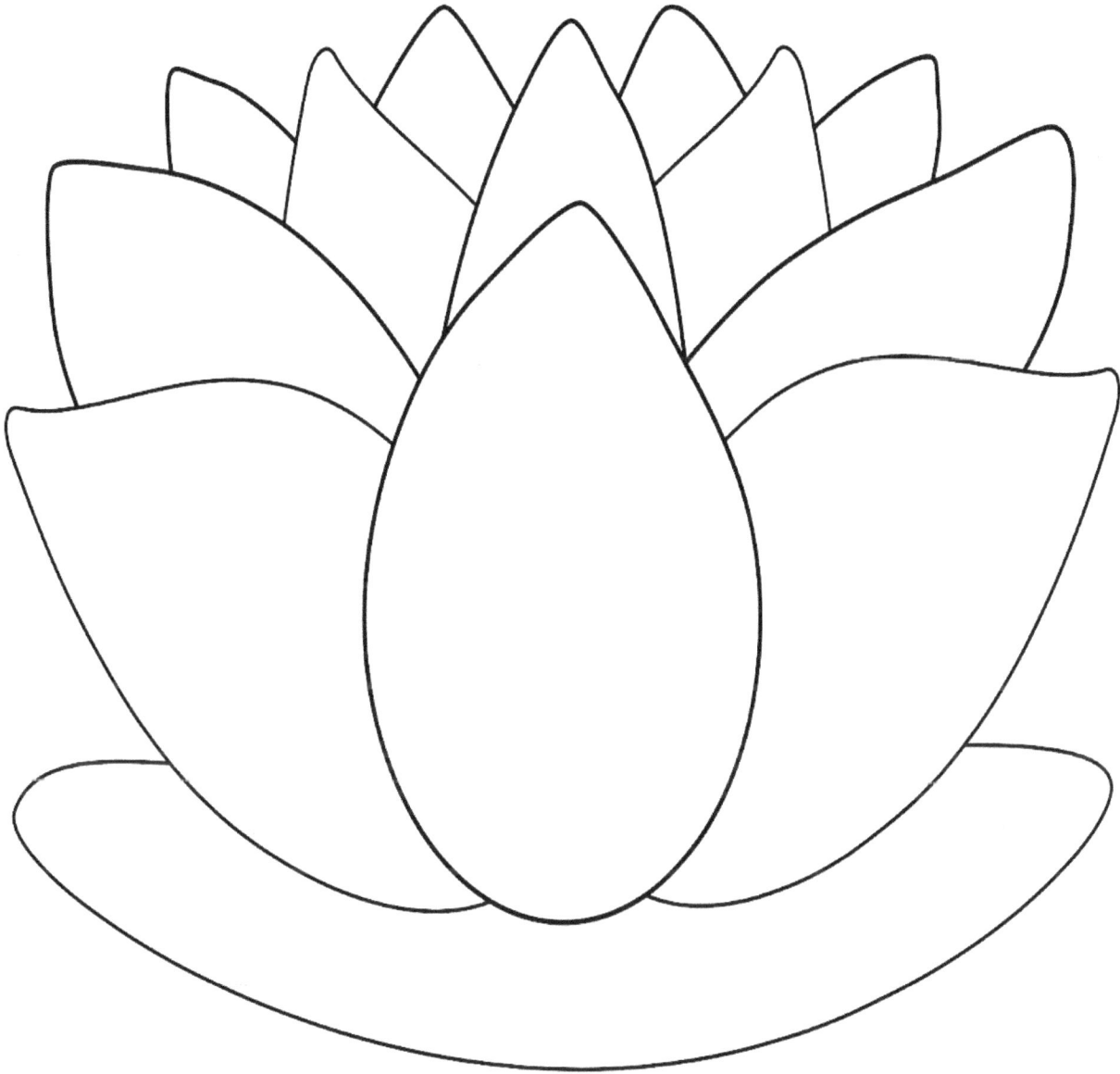

Day / Date : _____

Meal	Details	Calories
Breakfast		
Snack		
Lunch		
Snack		
Dinner		

Exercise	Time	Wt.	Sets/Reps
			/
			/
			/
			/
			/
			/
			/
			/
			/
			/
			/

Today's Results :

Blood Pressure / Time / Pulse :
/ __:__ _____
/ __:__ _____

Today's Weight :

Total Calories :

Water Intake :

Current Medications / Supplements :

What Inspired Me Today? (Ex: A Person, Goal Achieved, A Quote, or Misc.) :

My Progress Notes :

My Progress Reflections
& General Inspirations

_____

_____

_____

_____

_____

_____

_____

_____

_____

_____

_____

_____

_____

_____

_____

_____

Day / Date : _____

Meal	Details	Calories
Breakfast		
Snack		
Lunch		
Snack		
Dinner		

Exercise	Time	Wt.	Sets/Reps
			/
			/
			/
			/
			/
			/
			/
			/
			/
			/
			/
			/

Today's Results :

Blood Pressure / Time / Pulse :

/   __:__   _____

/   __:__   _____

Today's Weight :

Total Calories :

Water Intake :

Current Medications / Supplements :

What Inspired Me Today? (Ex: A Person, Goal Achieved, A Quote, or Misc.) :

_____

_____

_____

_____

My Progress Notes :

_____

_____

_____

_____

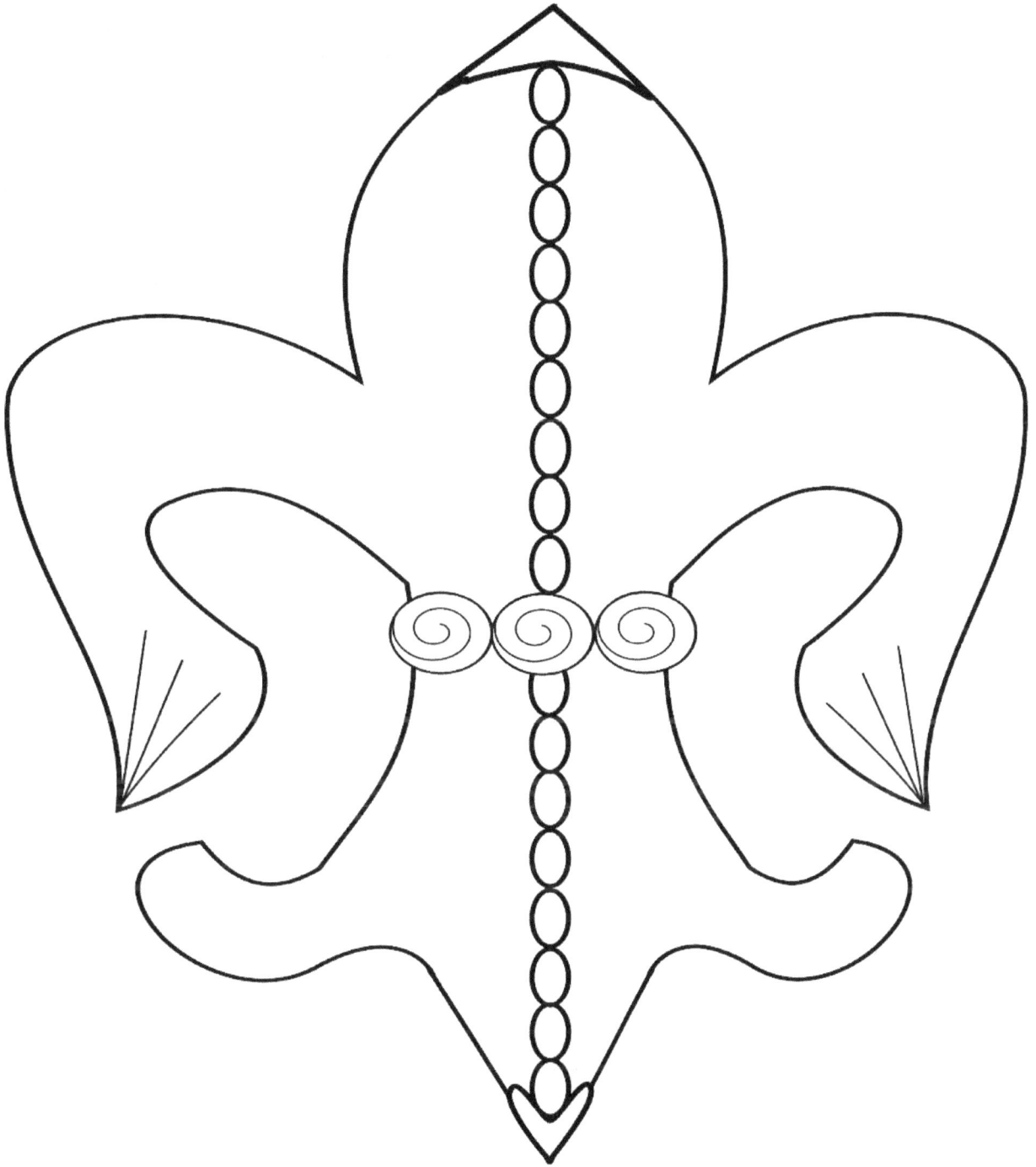

Day / Date : _____

Meal	Details	Calories
Breakfast		
Snack		
Lunch		
Snack		
Dinner		

Exercise	Time	Wt.	Sets/Reps
			/
			/
			/
			/
			/
			/
			/
			/
			/
			/
			/

Today's Results :

Blood Pressure /Time/Pulse :

/ __:__ _____

/ __:__ _____

Today's Weight :

Total Calories :

Water Intake :

Current Medications / Supplements :

What Inspired Me Today? (Ex: A Person, Goal Achieved, A Quote, or Misc.) :

_____
_____
_____
_____

My Progress Notes :

_____
_____
_____
_____

My Progress Reflections
& General Inspirations

_____

_____

_____

_____

_____

_____

_____

_____

_____

_____

_____

_____

_____

_____

_____

_____

_____

Day / Date : _____

Meal	Details	Calories
Breakfast		
Snack		
Lunch		
Snack		
Dinner		

Exercise	Time	Wt.	Sets/Reps
			/
			/
			/
			/
			/
			/
			/
			/
			/
			/
			/
			/

Today's Results :

Blood Pressure /Time/Pulse :
/ __:__ _____
/ __:__ _____

Today's Weight :

Total Calories :

Water Intake :

Current Medications / Supplements :

What Inspired Me Today? (Ex: A Person, Goal Achieved, A Quote, or Misc.) :

My Progress Notes :

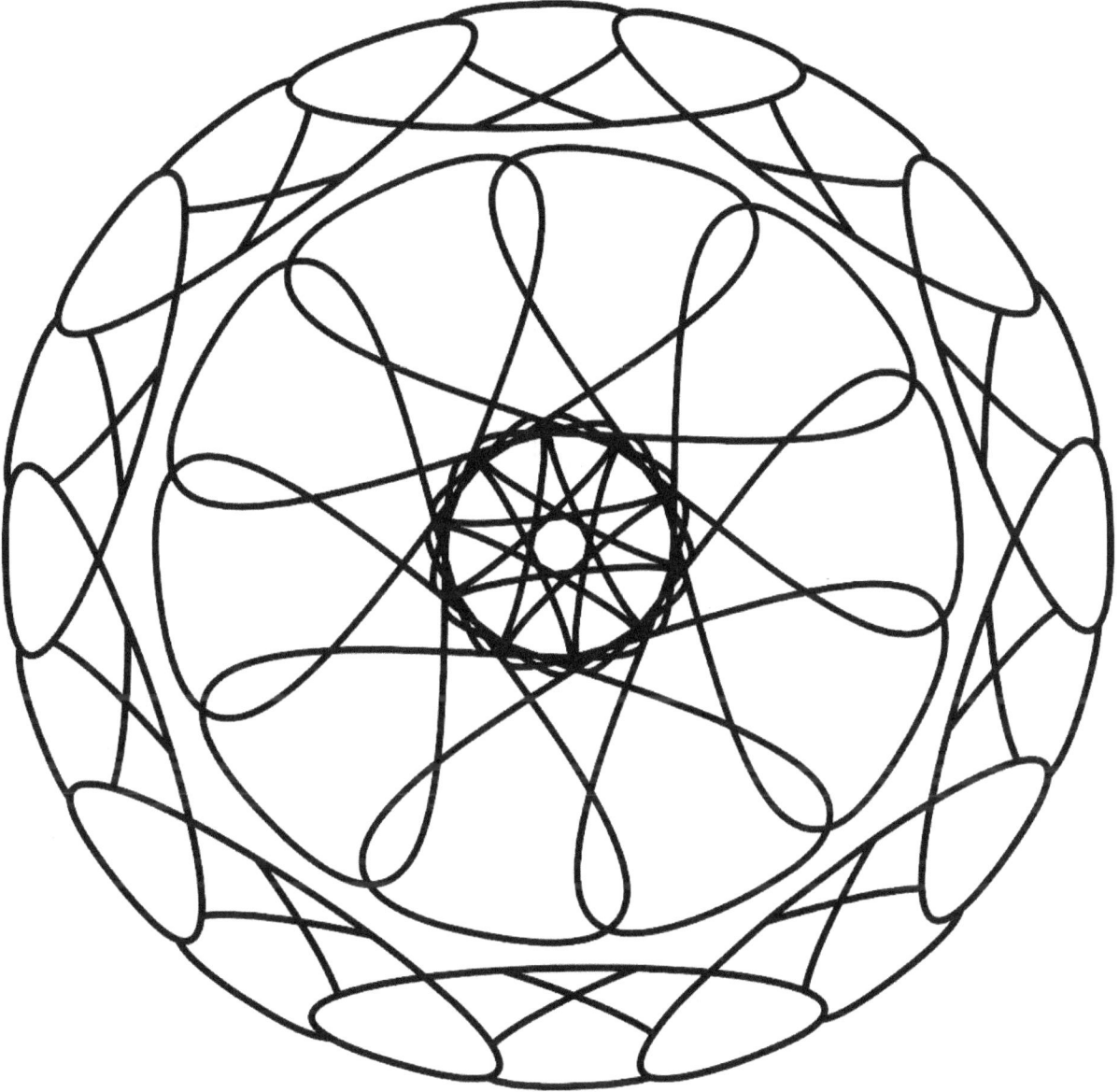

Day / Date : _____

Meal	Details	Calories
Breakfast		
Snack		
Lunch		
Snack		
Dinner		

Exercise	Time	Wt.	Sets/Reps
			/
			/
			/
			/
			/
			/
			/
			/
			/
			/
			/

Today's Results :

Blood Pressure / Time / Pulse :

/   __:__   _____

/   __:__   _____

Today's Weight :

Total Calories :

Water Intake :

Current Medications / Supplements :

What Inspired Me Today? (Ex: A Person, Goal Achieved, A Quote, or Misc.) :

My Progress Notes :

My Progress Reflections
& General Inspirations

_____

_____

_____

_____

_____

_____

_____

_____

_____

_____

_____

_____

_____

_____

_____

_____

_____

Day / Date : _____

Meal	Details	Calories
Breakfast		
Snack		
Lunch		
Snack		
Dinner		

Exercise	Time	Wt.	Sets/Reps
			/
			/
			/
			/
			/
			/
			/
			/
			/
			/
			/
			/

Today's Results :

Blood Pressure /Time/Pulse :

/ ___:___ _____

/ ___:___ _____

Today's Weight :

Total Calories :

Water Intake :

Current Medications / Supplements :

What Inspired Me Today? (Ex: A Person, Goal Achieved, A Quote, or Misc.) :

My Progress Notes :

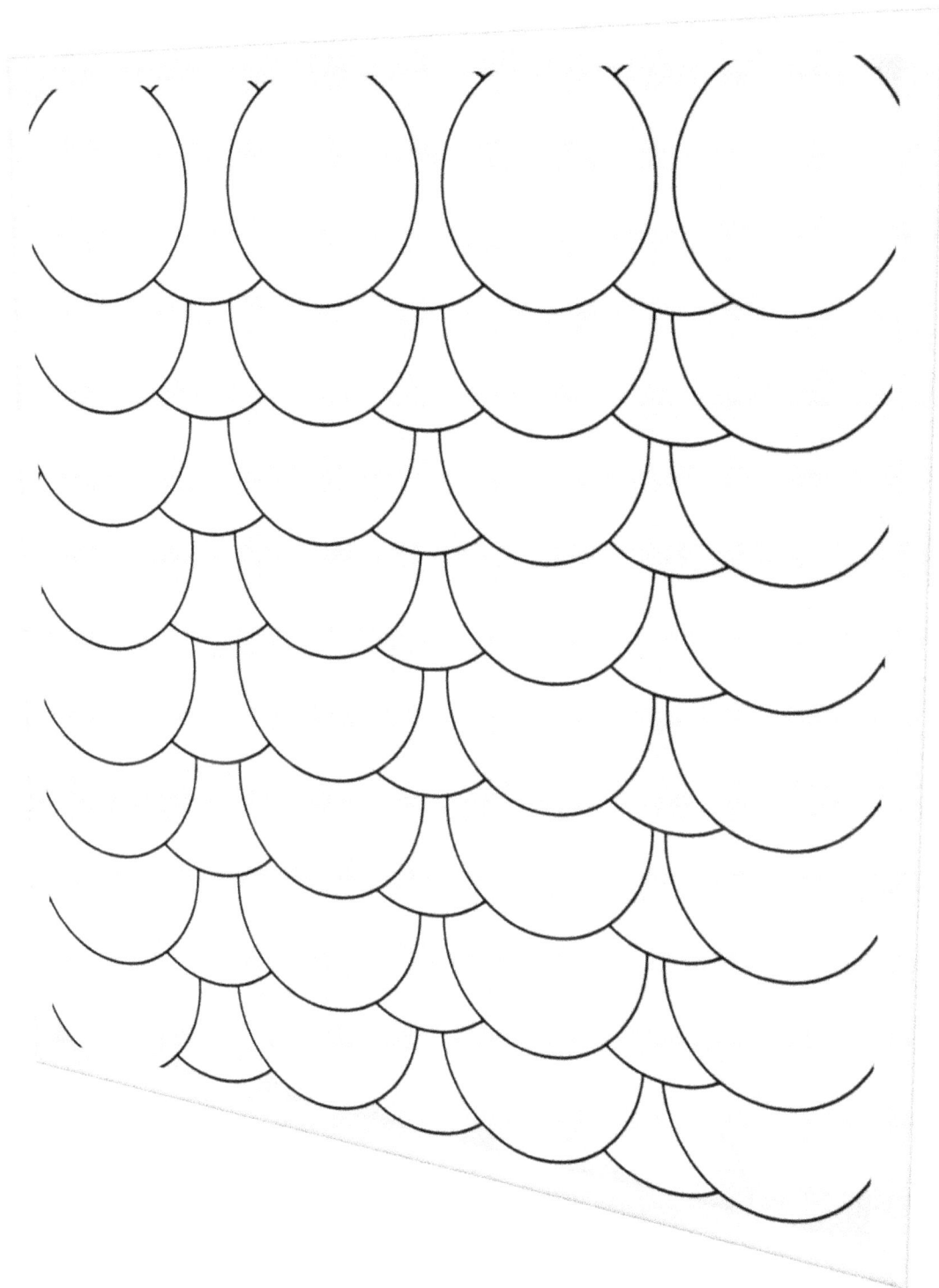

Day / Date : _____

Meal	Details	Calories
Breakfast		
Snack		
Lunch		
Snack		
Dinner		

Exercise	Time	Wt.	Sets/Reps
			/
			/
			/
			/
			/
			/
			/
			/
			/
			/
			/
			/

Today's Results :

Blood Pressure /Time/Pulse :

/ ___:___ _____

/ ___:___ _____

Today's Weight :

Total Calories :

Water Intake :

Current Medications / Supplements :

What Inspired Me Today? (Ex: A Person, Goal Achieved, A Quote, or Misc.) :

My Progress Notes :

My Progress Reflections
& General Inspirations

_____

_____

_____

_____

_____

_____

_____

_____

_____

_____

_____

_____

_____

_____

_____

_____

Day / Date : _____

Meal	Details	Calories
Breakfast		
Snack		
Lunch		
Snack		
Dinner		

Exercise	Time	Wt.	Sets/Reps
			/
			/
			/
			/
			/
			/
			/
			/
			/
			/
			/

Today's Results :

Blood Pressure /Time/Pulse :

/ ___:___ _____
/ ___:___ _____

Today's Weight :

Total Calories :

Water Intake :

Current Medications / Supplements :

What Inspired Me Today? (Ex: A Person, Goal Achieved, A Quote, or Misc.) :

My Progress Notes :

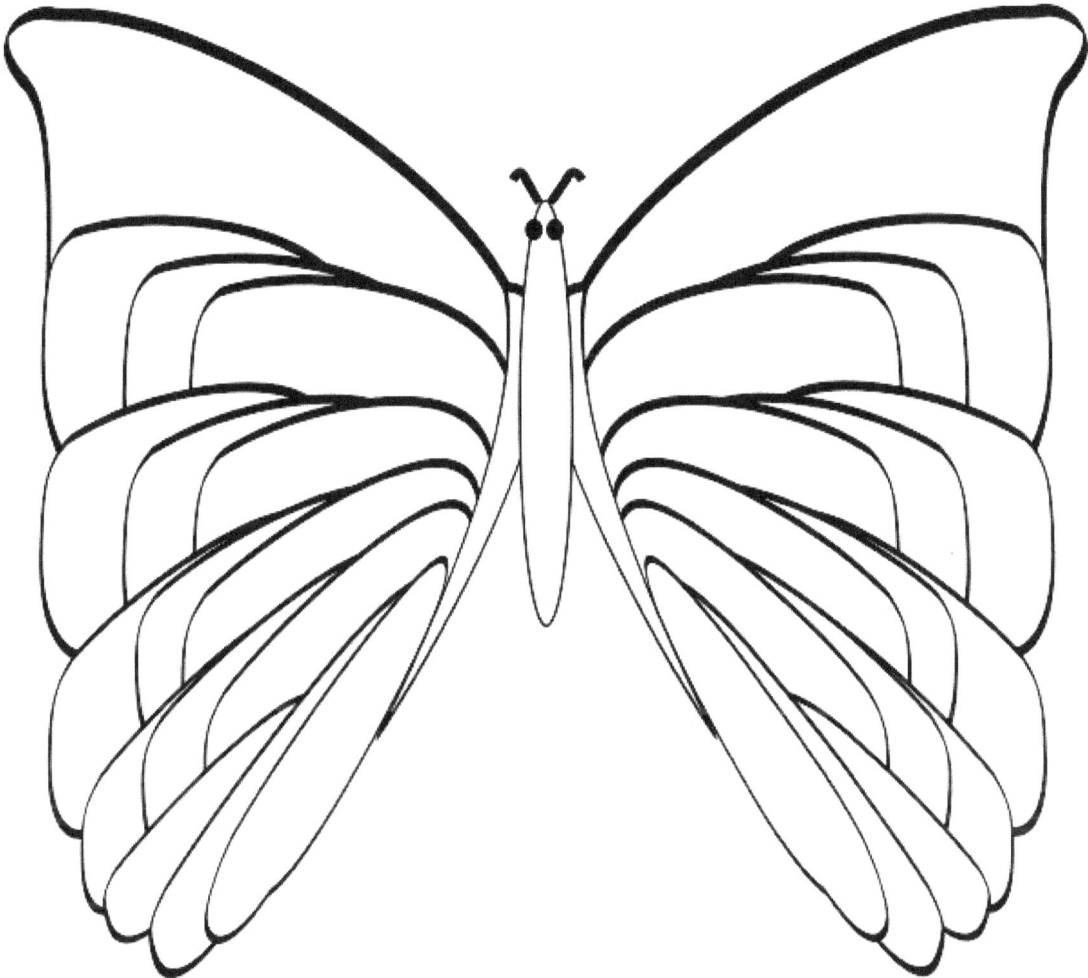

Day / Date : _____

Meal	Details	Calories
Breakfast		
Snack		
Lunch		
Snack		
Dinner		

Exercise	Time	Wt.	Sets/Reps
			/
			/
			/
			/
			/
			/
			/
			/
			/
			/
			/
			/

Today's Results :

Blood Pressure /Time/Pulse :
/ ___:___ _____
/ ___:___ _____

Today's Weight :

Total Calories :

Water Intake :

Current Medications / Supplements :

What Inspired Me Today? (Ex: A Person, Goal Achieved, A Quote, or Misc.) :

My Progress Notes :

My Progress Reflections
& General Inspirations

_____

_____

_____

_____

_____

_____

_____

_____

_____

_____

_____

_____

_____

_____

_____

_____

_____

Day / Date : _____

Meal	Details	Calories
Breakfast		
Snack		
Lunch		
Snack		
Dinner		

Exercise	Time	Wt.	Sets/Reps
			/
			/
			/
			/
			/
			/
			/
			/
			/
			/
			/

Today's Results :

Blood Pressure /Time/Pulse :
/ __:__ _____
/ __:__ _____

Today's Weight :

Total Calories :

Water Intake :

Current Medications / Supplements :

What Inspired Me Today? (Ex: A Person, Goal Achieved, A Quote, or Misc.) :

My Progress Notes :

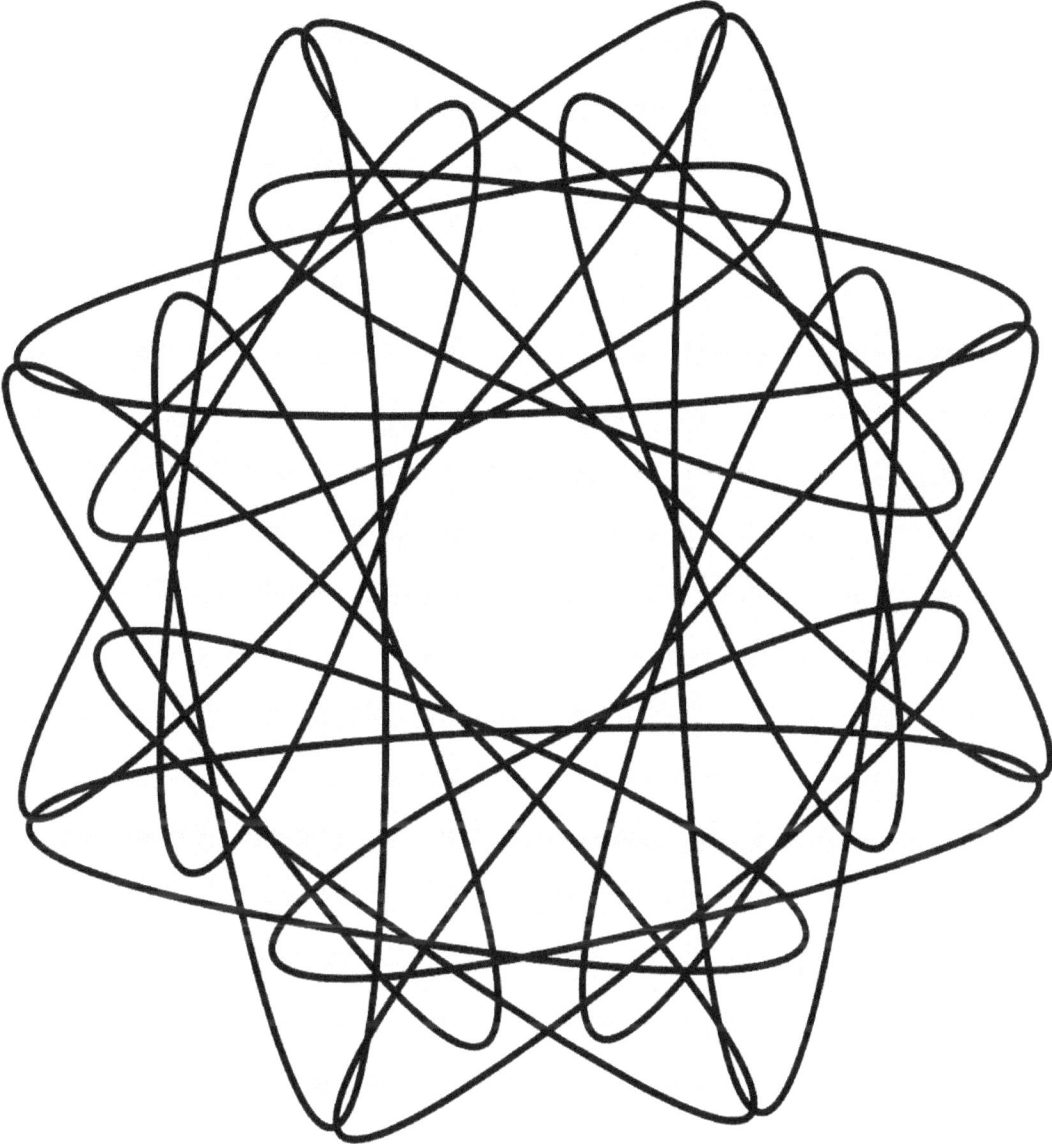

Day / Date : _____

Meal	Details	Calories
Breakfast		
Snack		
Lunch		
Snack		
Dinner		

Exercise	Time	Wt.	Sets/Reps
			/
			/
			/
			/
			/
			/
			/
			/
			/
			/
			/

Today's Results :

Blood Pressure /Time/Pulse :

/   __:__   _____
/   __:__   _____

Today's Weight :

Total Calories :

Water Intake :

Current Medications / Supplements :

What Inspired Me Today? (Ex: A Person, Goal Achieved, A Quote, or Misc.) :

My Progress Notes :

My Progress Reflections
& General Inspirations

_____

_____

_____

_____

_____

_____

_____

_____

_____

_____

_____

_____

_____

_____

_____

_____

_____

Day / Date : _____

Meal	Details	Calories
Breakfast		
Snack		
Lunch		
Snack		
Dinner		

Exercise	Time	Wt.	Sets/Reps
			/
			/
			/
			/
			/
			/
			/
			/
			/
			/
			/
			/

Today's Results :

Blood Pressure /Time/Pulse :
/ __:__ _____
/ __:__ _____

Today's Weight :

Total Calories :

Water Intake :

Current Medications / Supplements :

What Inspired Me Today? (Ex: A Person, Goal Achieved, A Quote, or Misc.) :

My Progress Notes :

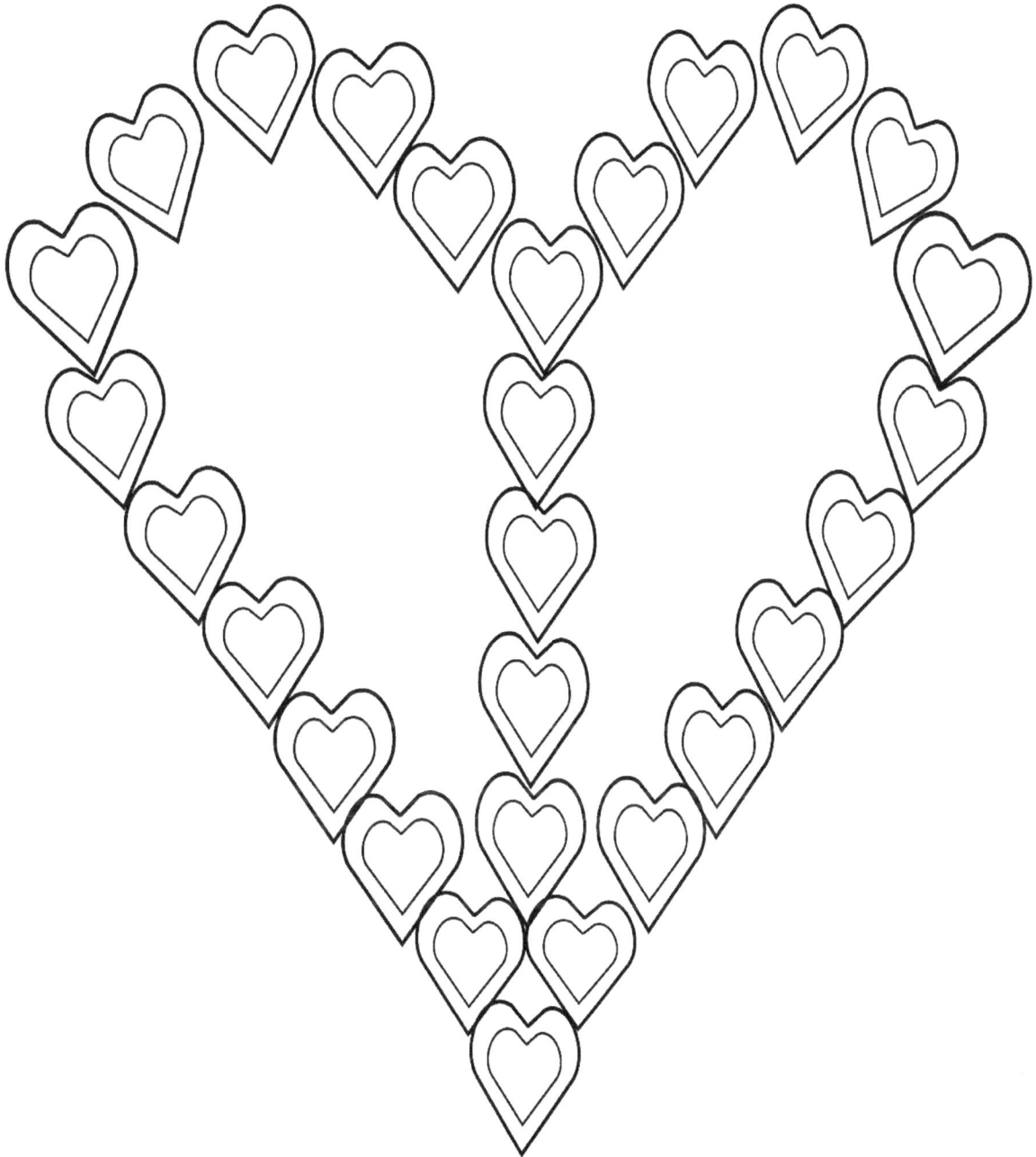

Day / Date : _____

Meal	Details	Calories
Breakfast		
Snack		
Lunch		
Snack		
Dinner		

Exercise	Time	Wt.	Sets/Reps
			/
			/
			/
			/
			/
			/
			/
			/
			/
			/
			/
			/

Today's Results :

Blood Pressure /Time/Pulse :

/ ___:___ _____

/ ___:___ _____

Today's Weight :

Total Calories :

Water Intake :

Current Medications / Supplements :

What Inspired Me Today? (Ex: A Person, Goal Achieved, A Quote, or Misc.) :

My Progress Notes :

My Progress Reflections & General Inspirations

_____

_____

_____

_____

_____

_____

_____

_____

_____

_____

_____

_____

_____

_____

_____

Day / Date : _____

Meal	Details	Calories
Breakfast		
Snack		
Lunch		
Snack		
Dinner		

Exercise	Time	Wt.	Sets/Reps
			/
			/
			/
			/
			/
			/
			/
			/
			/
			/
			/
			/

Today's Results :

Blood Pressure /Time/Pulse :
/   __:__   _____
/   __:__   _____

Today's Weight :

Total Calories :

Water Intake :

Current Medications / Supplements :

What Inspired Me Today? (Ex: A Person, Goal Achieved, A Quote, or Misc.) :

My Progress Notes :

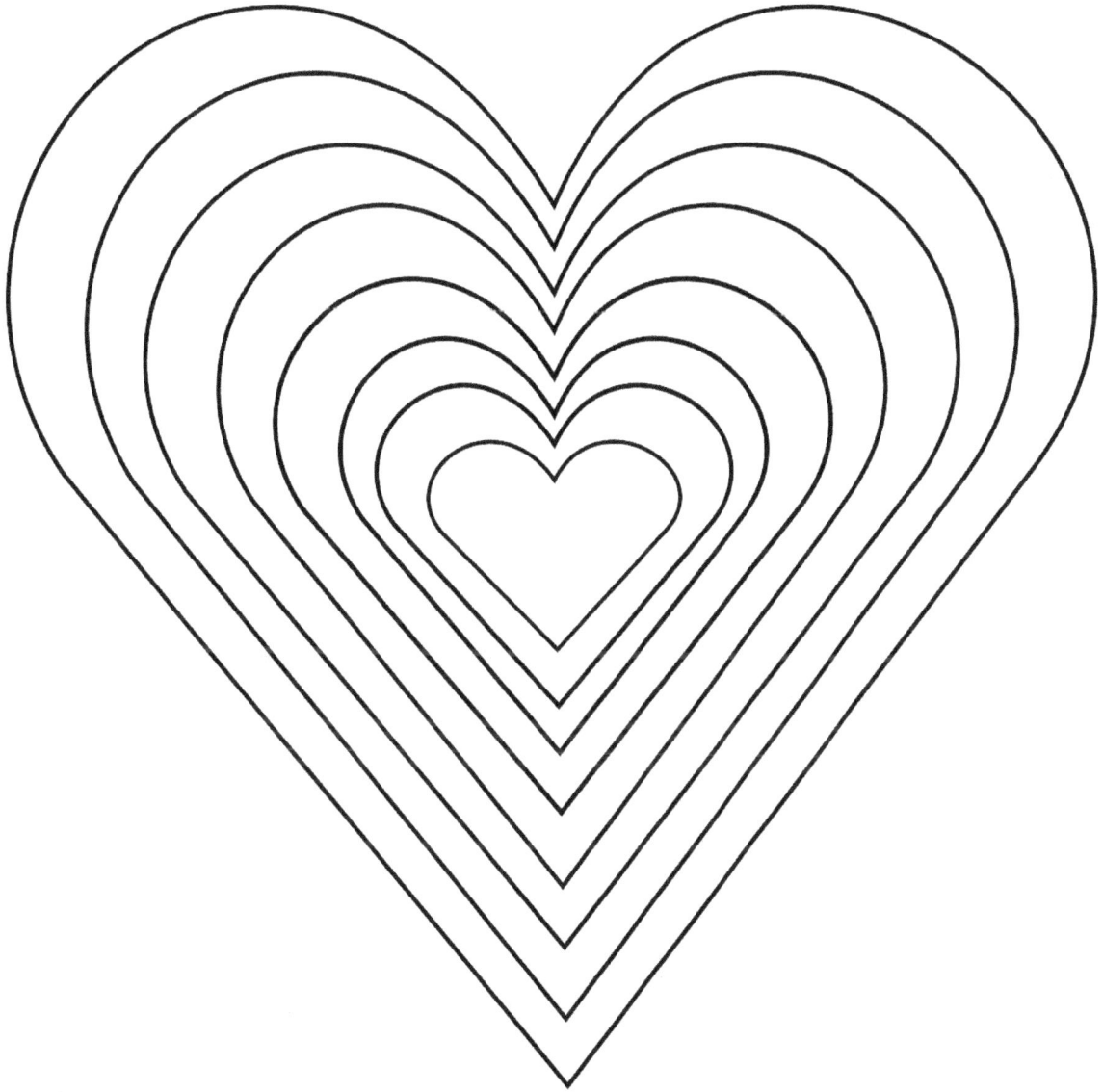

Day / Date : _____

Meal	Details	Calories
Breakfast		
Snack		
Lunch		
Snack		
Dinner		

Today's Results :

Blood Pressure /Time/Pulse :

/   __:__   _____

/   __:__   _____

Today's Weight :

Total Calories :

Water Intake :

Current Medications / Supplements :

Exercise	Time	Wt.	Sets/Reps
			/
			/
			/
			/
			/
			/
			/
			/
			/
			/
			/

What Inspired Me Today? (Ex: A Person, Goal Achieved, A Quote, or Misc.) :

My Progress Notes :

My Progress Reflections
& General Inspirations

_____

_____

_____

_____

_____

_____

_____

_____

_____

_____

_____

_____

_____

_____

_____

_____

Day / Date : _____

Meal	Details	Calories		Exercise	Time	Wt.	Sets/Reps
Breakfast							/
Snack							/
Lunch							/
Snack							/
Dinner							/
							/
							/
							/
							/
							/
							/
							/

Today's Results :

Blood Pressure /Time/Pulse :
/ ___:___ _____
/ ___:___ _____

Today's Weight :

Total Calories :

Water Intake :

Current Medications / Supplements :

What Inspired Me Today? (Ex: A Person, Goal Achieved, A Quote, or Misc.) :

My Progress Notes :

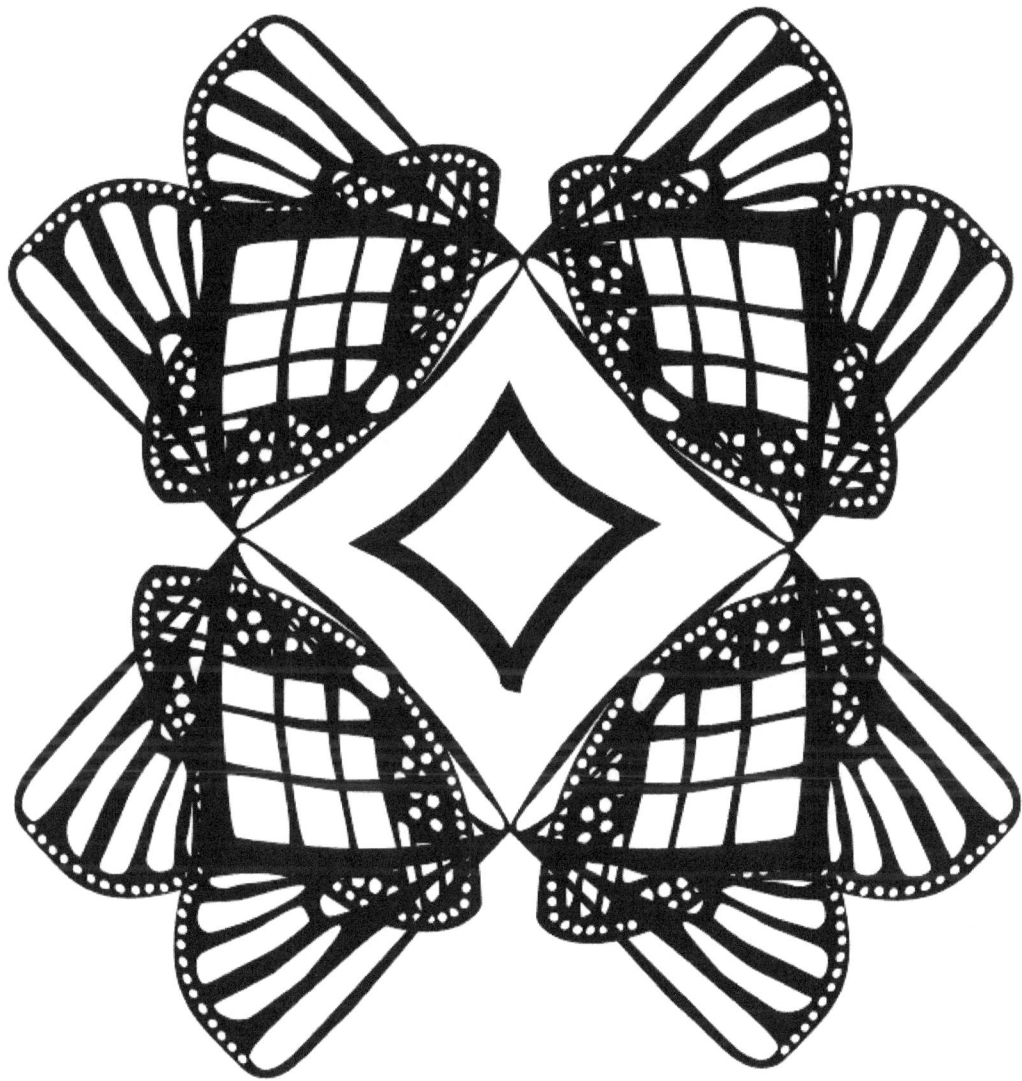

Day / Date : _____

Meal	Details	Calories
Breakfast		
Snack		
Lunch		
Snack		
Dinner		

Exercise	Time	Wt.	Sets/Reps
			/
			/
			/
			/
			/
			/
			/
			/
			/
			/
			/

Today's Results :

Blood Pressure /Time/Pulse :

/ ___:___ _____

/ ___:___ _____

Today's Weight :

Total Calories :

Water Intake :

Current Medications / Supplements :

What Inspired Me Today? (Ex: A Person, Goal Achieved, A Quote, or Misc.) :

My Progress Notes :

My Progress Reflections
& General Inspirations

_____

_____

_____

_____

_____

_____

_____

_____

_____

_____

_____

_____

_____

_____

_____

_____

Day / Date : _____

Meal	Details	Calories
Breakfast		
Snack		
Lunch		
Snack		
Dinner		

Exercise	Time	Wt.	Sets/Reps
			/
			/
			/
			/
			/
			/
			/
			/
			/
			/
			/

Today's Results :

Blood Pressure /Time/Pulse :
/   __:__   _____
/   __:__   _____

Today's Weight :

Total Calories :

Water Intake :

Current Medications / Supplements :

What Inspired Me Today? (Ex: A Person, Goal Achieved, A Quote, or Misc.) :

My Progress Notes :

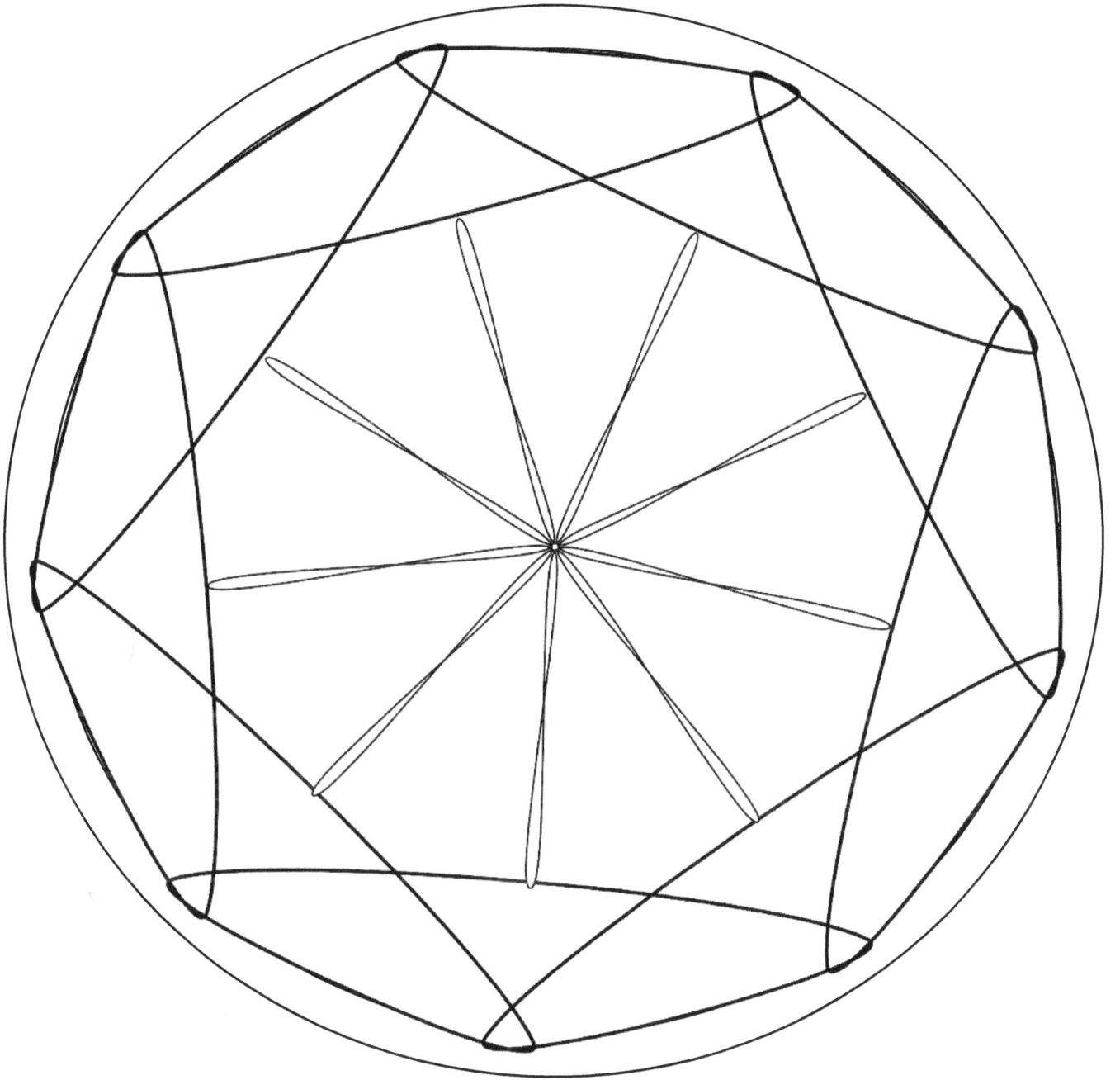

Day / Date : _____

Meal	Details	Calories
Breakfast		
Snack		
Lunch		
Snack		
Dinner		

Exercise	Time	Wt.	Sets/Reps
			/
			/
			/
			/
			/
			/
			/
			/
			/
			/
			/
			/

Today's Results :

Blood Pressure /Time/Pulse :

/ ___:___ _____
/ ___:___ _____

Today's Weight :

Total Calories :

Water Intake :

Current Medications / Supplements :

What Inspired Me Today? (Ex: A Person, Goal Achieved, A Quote, or Misc.) :

My Progress Notes :

My Progress Reflections & General Inspirations

_____

_____

_____

_____

_____

_____

_____

_____

_____

_____

_____

_____

_____

_____

_____

_____

_____

Day / Date : _____

Meal	Details	Calories
Breakfast		
Snack		
Lunch		
Snack		
Dinner		

Exercise	Time	Wt.	Sets/Reps
			/
			/
			/
			/
			/
			/
			/
			/
			/
			/
			/

Today's Results :

Blood Pressure /Time/Pulse :

/   __:__   _____
/   __:__   _____

Today's Weight :

Total Calories :

Water Intake :

Current Medications / Supplements :

What Inspired Me Today? (Ex: A Person, Goal Achieved, A Quote, or Misc.) :

My Progress Notes :

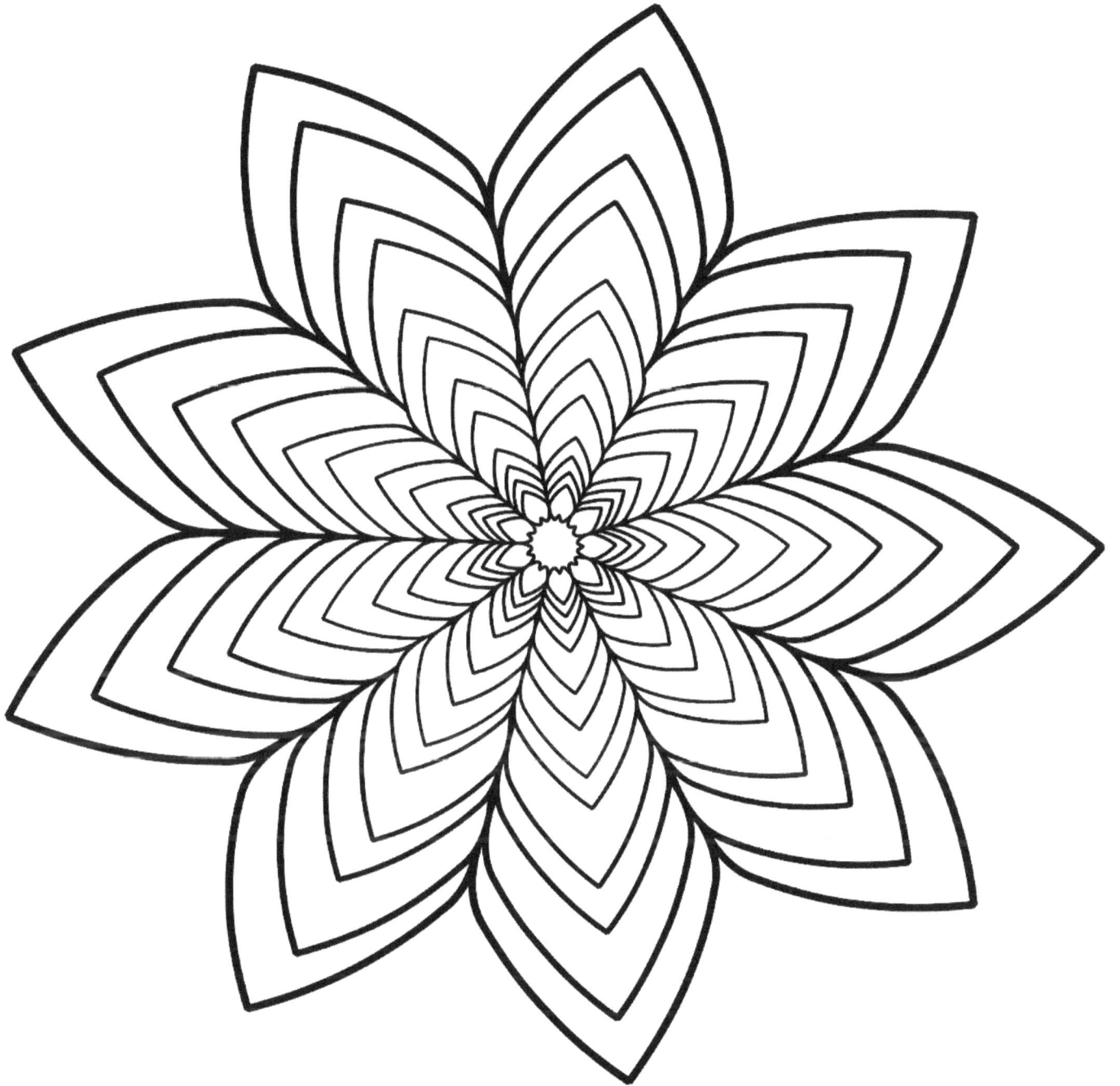

Day / Date : _____

Meal	Details	Calories
Breakfast		
Snack		
Lunch		
Snack		
Dinner		

Exercise	Time	Wt.	Sets/Reps
			/
			/
			/
			/
			/
			/
			/
			/
			/
			/
			/

Today's Results :

Blood Pressure /Time/Pulse :

/   __:__   _____
/   __:__   _____

Today's Weight :

Total Calories :

Water Intake :

Current Medications / Supplements :

What Inspired Me Today? (Ex: A Person, Goal Achieved, A Quote, or Misc.) :

My Progress Notes :

My Progress Reflections & General Inspirations

_____

_____

_____

_____

_____

_____

_____

_____

_____

_____

_____

_____

_____

_____

Day / Date : _____

Meal	Details	Calories
Breakfast		
Snack		
Lunch		
Snack		
Dinner		

Exercise	Time	Wt.	Sets/Reps
			/
			/
			/
			/
			/
			/
			/
			/
			/
			/
			/
			/

Today's Results :

Blood Pressure / Time / Pulse :

/ ___:___ _____

/ ___:___ _____

Today's Weight :

Total Calories :

Water Intake :

Current Medications / Supplements :

What Inspired Me Today? (Ex: A Person, Goal Achieved, A Quote, or Misc.) :

My Progress Notes :

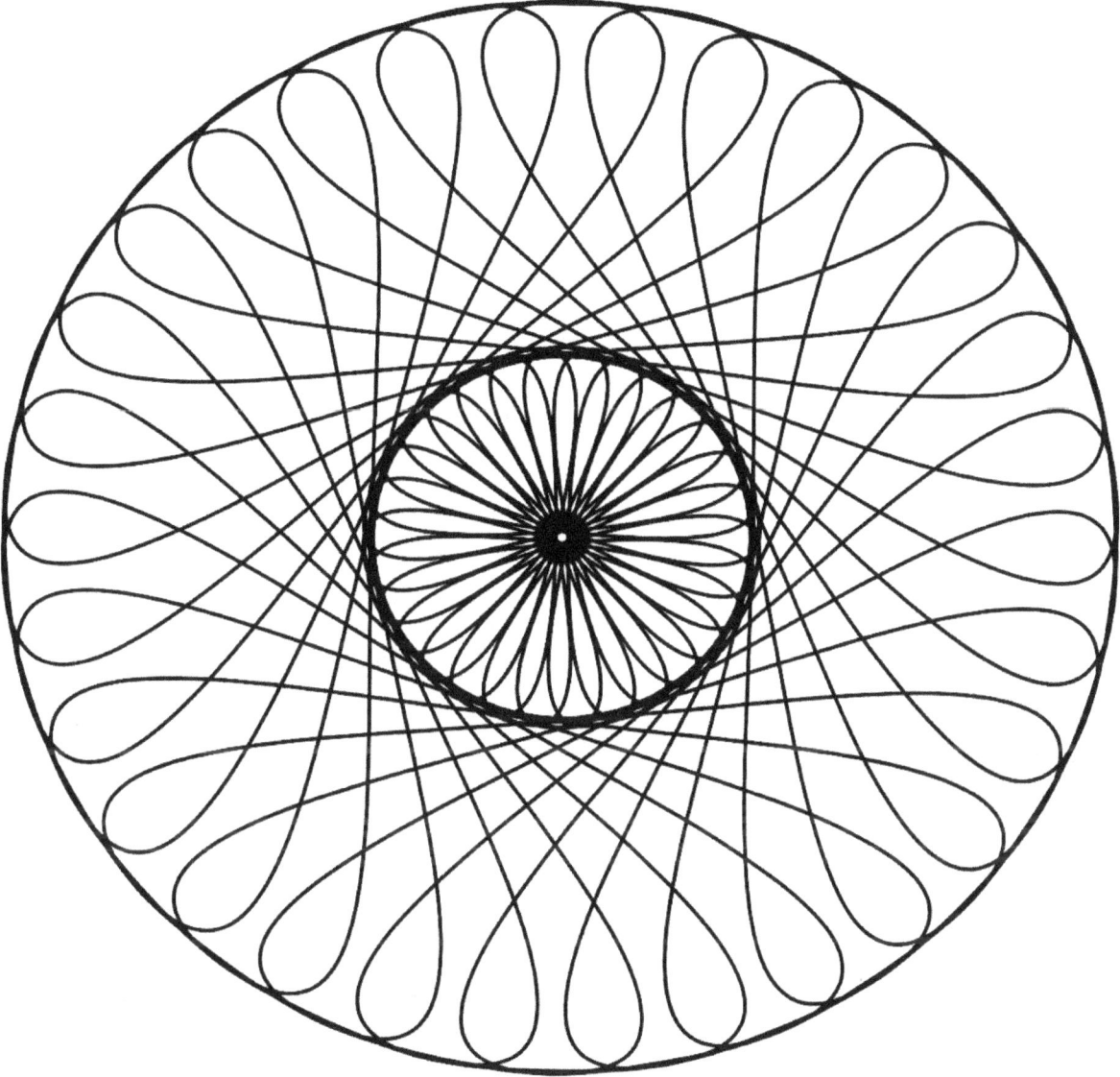

Day / Date : _____

Meal	Details	Calories
Breakfast		
Snack		
Lunch		
Snack		
Dinner		

Exercise	Time	Wt.	Sets/Reps
			/
			/
			/
			/
			/
			/
			/
			/
			/
			/
			/

Today's Results :

Blood Pressure /Time/Pulse :

/ ____:____ _____

/ ____:____ _____

Today's Weight :

Total Calories :

Water Intake :

Current Medications / Supplements :

What Inspired Me Today? (Ex: A Person, Goal Achieved, A Quote, or Misc.) :

My Progress Notes :

My Progress Reflections
& General Inspirations

_____

_____

_____

_____

_____

_____

_____

_____

_____

_____

_____

_____

_____

_____

_____

_____

Day / Date : _____

Meal	Details	Calories
Breakfast		
Snack		
Lunch		
Snack		
Dinner		

Exercise	Time	Wt.	Sets/Reps
			/
			/
			/
			/
			/
			/
			/
			/
			/
			/
			/

Today's Results :

Blood Pressure /Time/Pulse :

    /   __:__   _____

    /   __:__   _____

Today's Weight :

Total Calories :

Water Intake :

Current Medications / Supplements :

What Inspired Me Today? (Ex. A Person, Goal Achieved, A Quote, or Misc.) :

_____

_____

_____

_____

My Progress Notes :

_____

_____

_____

_____

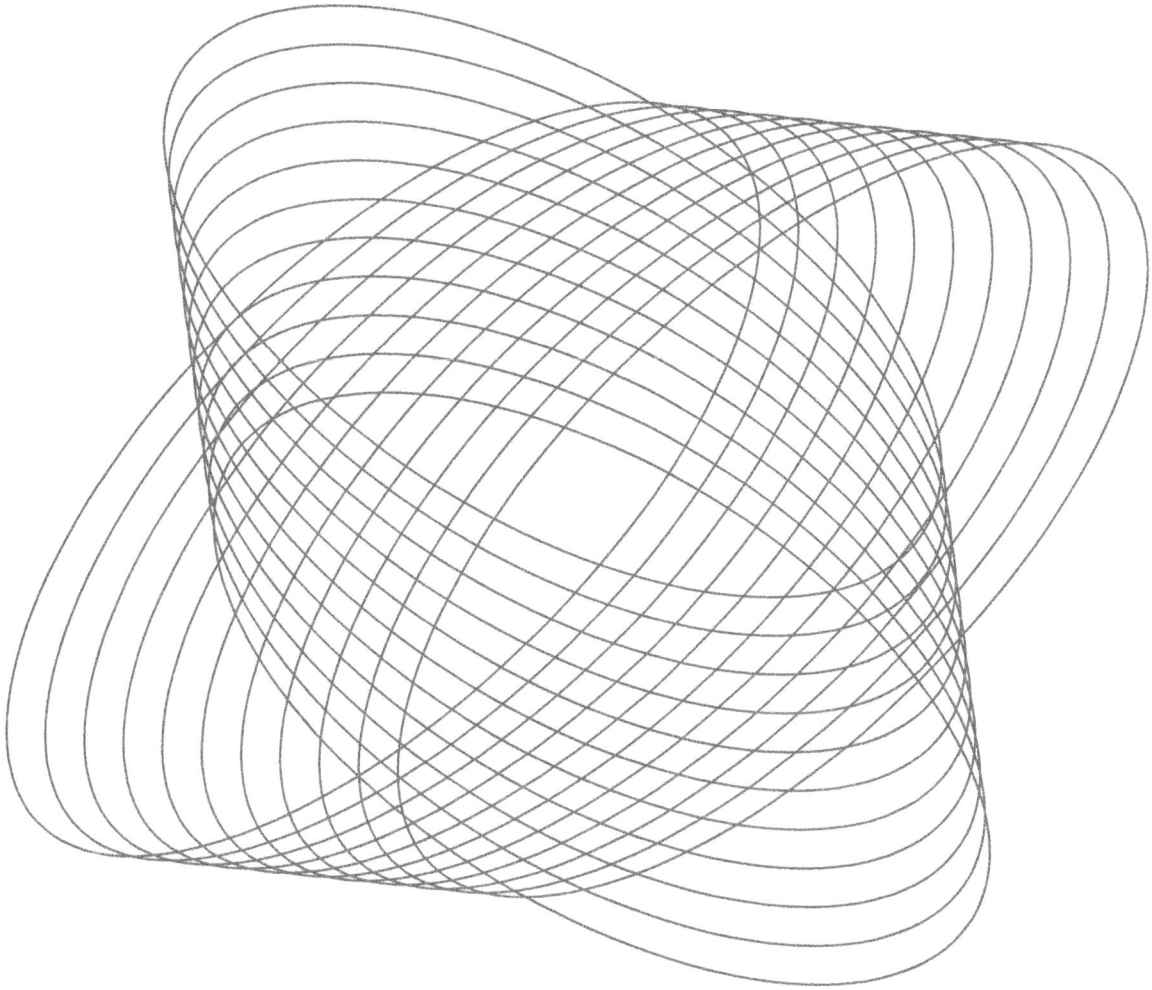

Day / Date : _____

Meal	Details	Calories
Breakfast		
Snack		
Lunch		
Snack		
Dinner		

Exercise	Time	Wt.	Sets/Reps
			/
			/
			/
			/
			/
			/
			/
			/
			/
			/
			/

Today's Results :

Blood Pressure /Time/Pulse :

/ ___:___ _____

/ ___:___ _____

Today's Weight :

Total Calories :

Water Intake :

Current Medications / Supplements :

What Inspired Me Today? (Ex: A Person, Goal Achieved, A Quote, or Misc.) :

My Progress Notes :

My Progress Reflections
& General Inspirations

_____

_____

_____

_____

_____

_____

_____

_____

_____

_____

_____

_____

_____

_____

_____

_____

Day / Date : _____

Meal	Details	Calories
Breakfast		
Snack		
Lunch		
Snack		
Dinner		

Exercise	Time	Wt.	Sets/Reps
			/
			/
			/
			/
			/
			/
			/
			/
			/
			/
			/
			/

Today's Results :

Blood Pressure / Time / Pulse :

/   __:__   _____

/   __:__   _____

Today's Weight :

Total Calories :

Water Intake :

Current Medications / Supplements :

What Inspired Me Today? (Ex: A Person, Goal Achieved, A Quote, or Misc.) :

_____

_____

_____

_____

My Progress Notes :

_____

_____

_____

_____

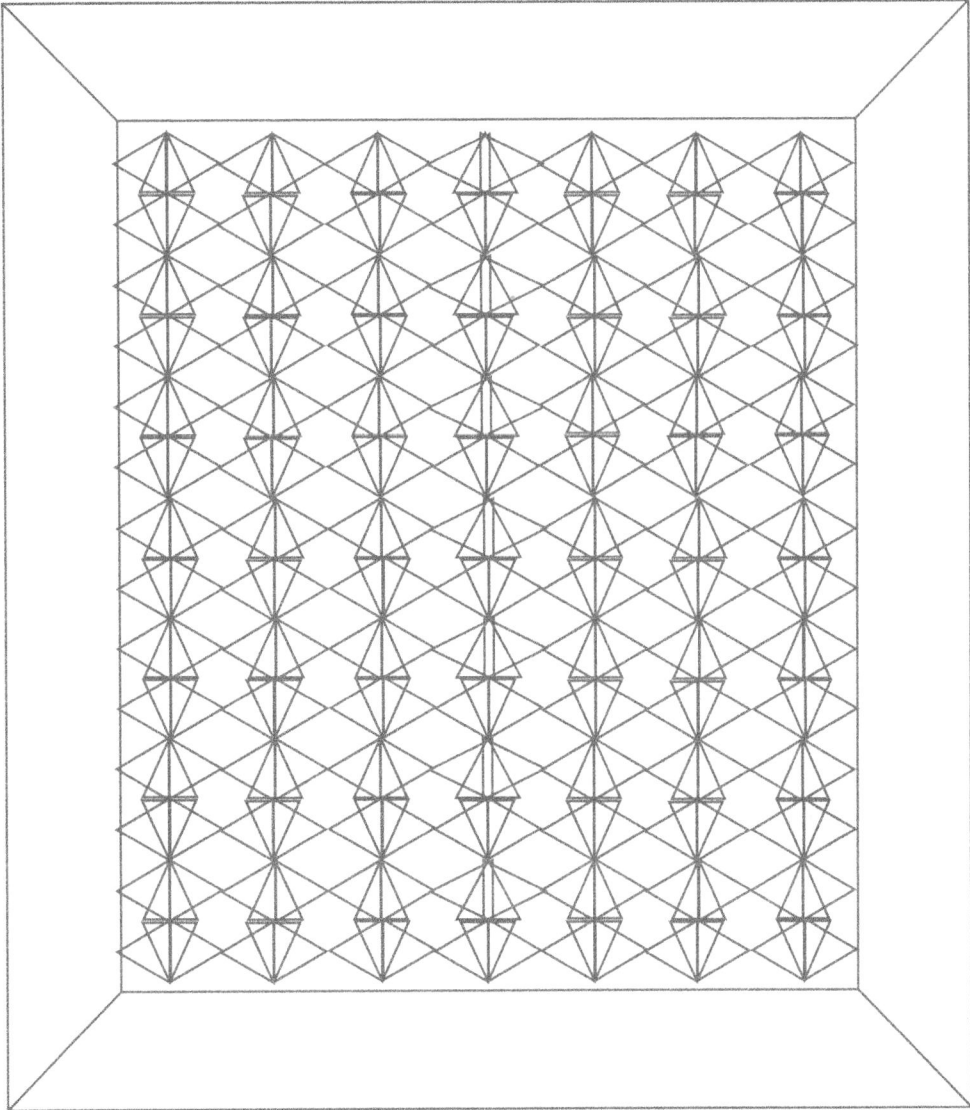

Day / Date : _____

Meal	Details	Calories
Breakfast		
Snack		
Lunch		
Snack		
Dinner		

Exercise	Time	Wt.	Sets/Reps
			/
			/
			/
			/
			/
			/
			/
			/
			/
			/
			/

Today's Results :

Blood Pressure /Time/Pulse :

/   __:__   _____
/   __:__   _____

Today's Weight :

Total Calories :

Water Intake :

Current Medications / Supplements :

What Inspired Me Today? (Ex: A Person, Goal Achieved, A Quote, or Misc.) :

My Progress Notes :

My Progress Reflections
& General Inspirations

_____

_____

_____

_____

_____

_____

_____

_____

_____

_____

_____

_____

_____

_____

_____

_____

_____

Day / Date : _____

Meal	Details	Calories
Breakfast		
Snack		
Lunch		
Snack		
Dinner		

Exercise	Time	Wt.	Sets/Reps
			/
			/
			/
			/
			/
			/
			/
			/
			/
			/
			/
			/

Today's Results :

Blood Pressure /Time/Pulse :

/   __:__   _____

/   __:__   _____

Today's Weight :

Total Calories :

Water Intake :

Current Medications / Supplements :

What Inspired Me Today? (Ex: A Person, Goal Achieved, A Quote, or Misc.) :

My Progress Notes :

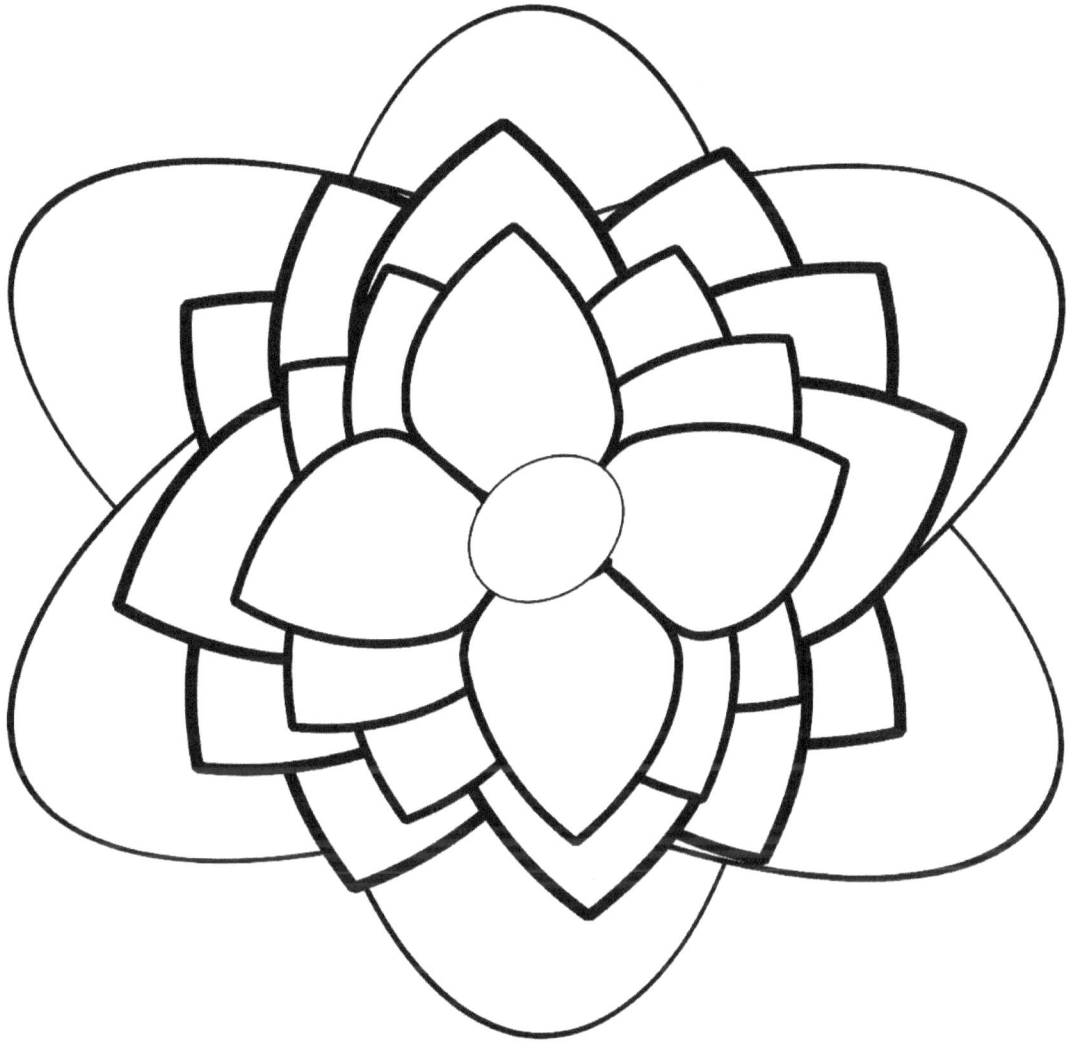

Day / Date : _____

Meal	Details	Calories
Breakfast		
Snack		
Lunch		
Snack		
Dinner		

Exercise	Time	Wt.	Sets/Reps
			/
			/
			/
			/
			/
			/
			/
			/
			/
			/
			/
			/

Today's Results :

Blood Pressure /Time/Pulse :

/   __:__   _____

/   __:__   _____

Today's Weight :

Total Calories :

Water Intake :

Current Medications / Supplements :

What Inspired Me Today? (Ex: A Person, Goal Achieved, A Quote, or Misc.) :

My Progress Notes :

My Progress Reflections
& General Inspirations

_____

_____

_____

_____

_____

_____

_____

_____

_____

_____

_____

_____

_____

_____

_____

_____

_____

Day / Date : _____

Meal	Details	Calories
Breakfast		
Snack		
Lunch		
Snack		
Dinner		

Exercise	Time	Wt.	Sets/Reps
			/
			/
			/
			/
			/
			/
			/
			/
			/
			/
			/
			/

Today's Results :

Blood Pressure / Time / Pulse :

/ __:__ _____
/ __:__ _____

Today's Weight :

Total Calories :

Water Intake :

Current Medications / Supplements :

What Inspired Me Today? (Ex: A Person, Goal Achieved, A Quote, or Misc.) :

_____

_____

_____

_____

My Progress Notes :

_____

_____

_____

_____

_____

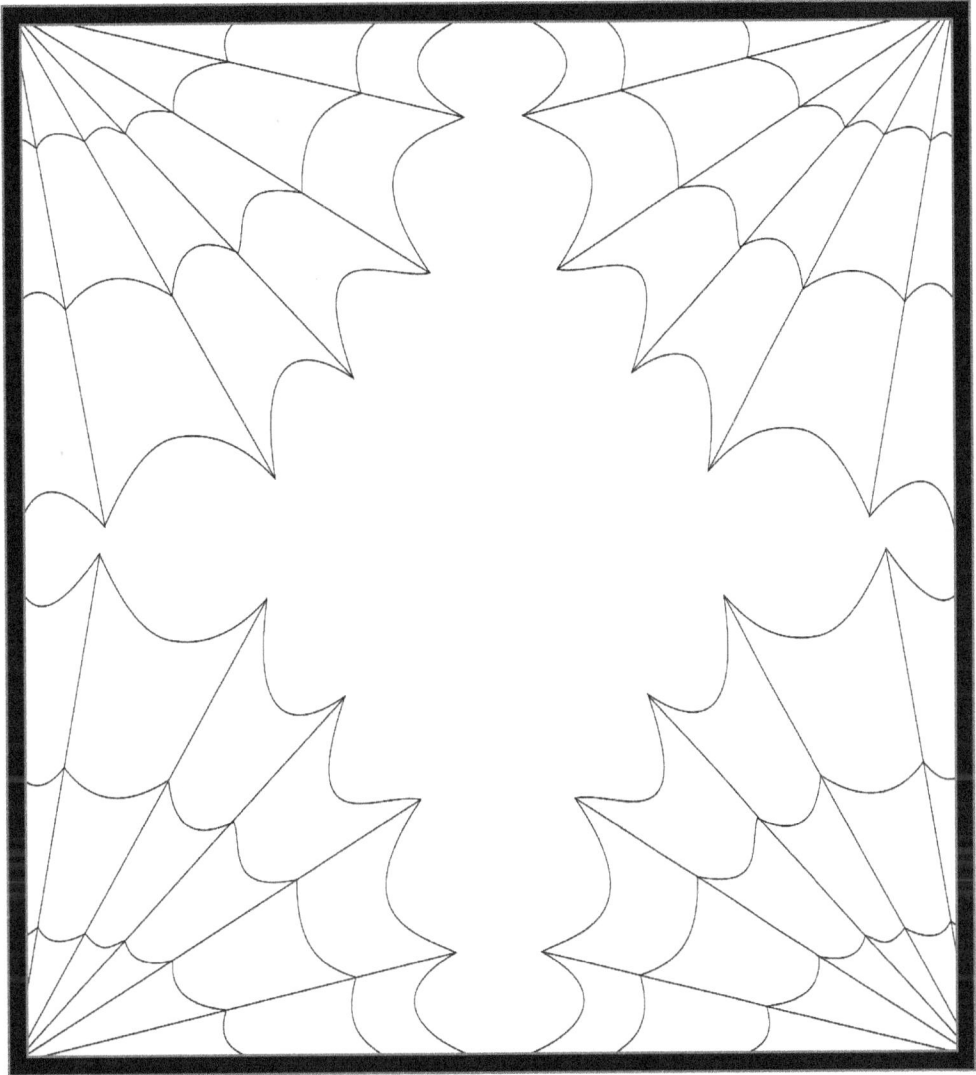

Day / Date : _____

Meal	Details	Calories
Breakfast		
Snack		
Lunch		
Snack		
Dinner		

Exercise	Time	Wt.	Sets/Reps
			/
			/
			/
			/
			/
			/
			/
			/
			/
			/
			/
			/

Today's Results :

Blood Pressure /Time/Pulse :

   /   __:__   _____

   /   __:__   _____

Today's Weight :

Total Calories :

Water Intake :

Current Medications / Supplements :

What Inspired Me Today? (Ex: A Person, Goal Achieved, A Quote, or Misc.) :

My Progress Notes :

My Progress Reflections
& General Inspirations

_____

_____

_____

_____

_____

_____

_____

_____

_____

_____

_____

_____

_____

_____

_____

_____

Day / Date : _____

Meal	Details	Calories
Breakfast		
Snack		
Lunch		
Snack		
Dinner		

Exercise	Time	Wt.	Sets/Reps
			/
			/
			/
			/
			/
			/
			/
			/
			/
			/
			/
			/

Today's Results :

Blood Pressure /Time/Pulse :

/   __:__   _____

/   __:__   _____

Today's Weight :

Total Calories :

Water Intake :

Current Medications / Supplements :

What Inspired Me Today? (Ex: A Person, Goal Achieved, A Quote, or Misc.) :

My Progress Notes :

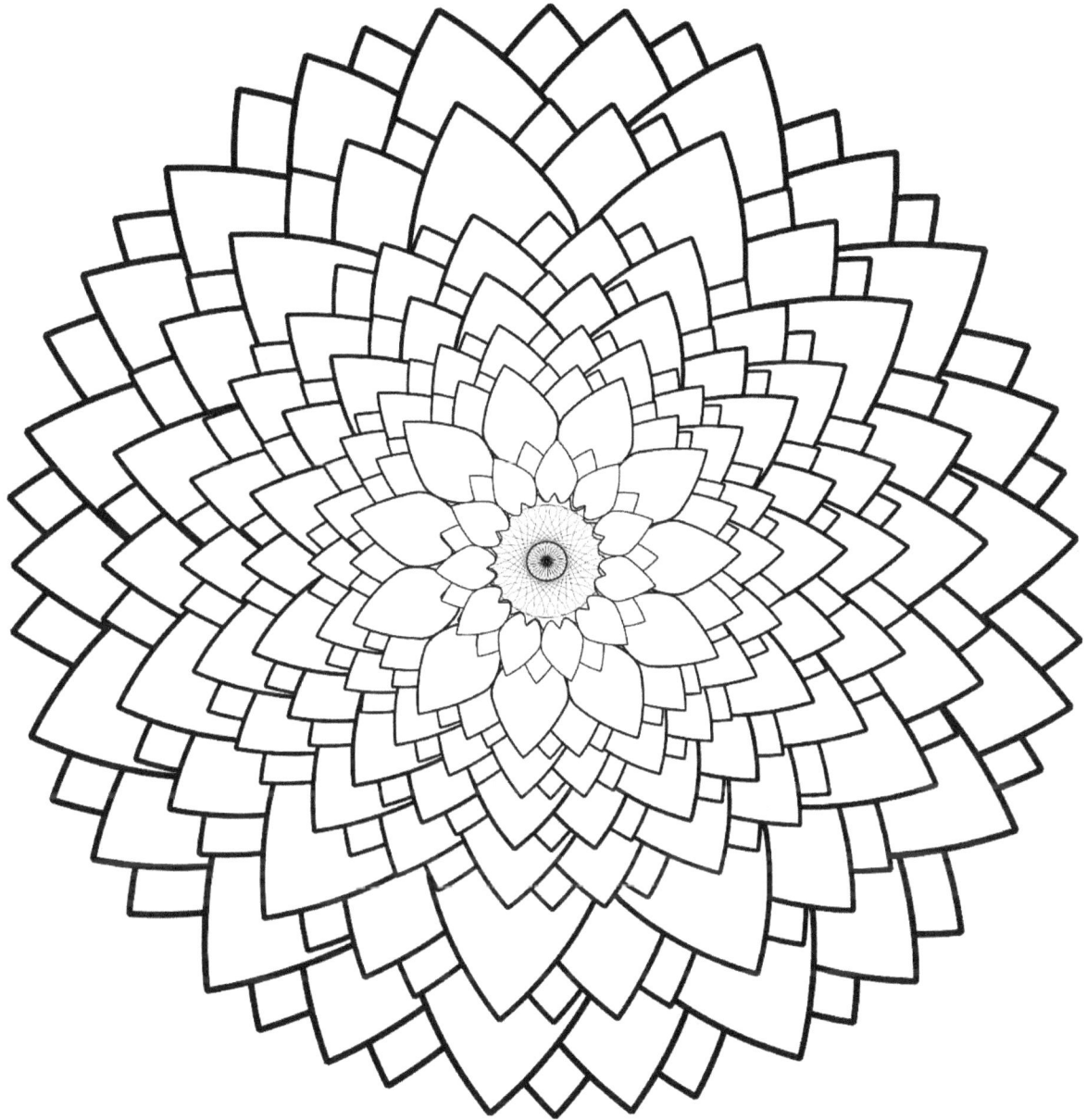

Day / Date : _____

Meal	Details	Calories
Breakfast		
Snack		
Lunch		
Snack		
Dinner		

Exercise	Time	Wt.	Sets/Reps
			/
			/
			/
			/
			/
			/
			/
			/
			/
			/
			/

Today's Results :

Blood Pressure /Time/Pulse :

   /   __:__   _____

   /   __:__   _____

Today's Weight :

Total Calories :

Water Intake :

Current Medications / Supplements :

What Inspired Me Today? (Ex: A Person, Goal Achieved, A Quote, or Misc.) :

My Progress Notes :

My Progress Reflections
& General Inspirations

_____

_____

_____

_____

_____

_____

_____

_____

_____

_____

_____

_____

_____

_____

_____

_____

Day / Date : _____

Meal	Details	Calories
Breakfast		
Snack		
Lunch		
Snack		
Dinner		

Exercise	Time	Wt.	Sets/Reps
			/
			/
			/
			/
			/
			/
			/
			/
			/
			/
			/

Today's Results :

Blood Pressure /Time/Pulse :

/   __:__   _____

/   __:__   _____

Today's Weight :

Total Calories :

Water Intake :

Current Medications / Supplements :

What Inspired Me Today? (Ex: A Person, Goal Achieved, A Quote, or Misc.) :

_____

_____

_____

_____

My Progress Notes :

_____

_____

_____

_____

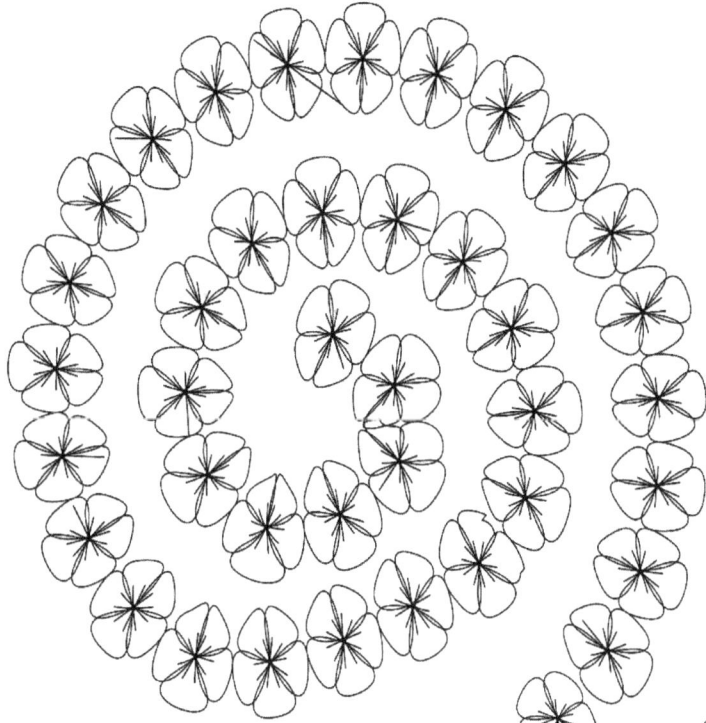

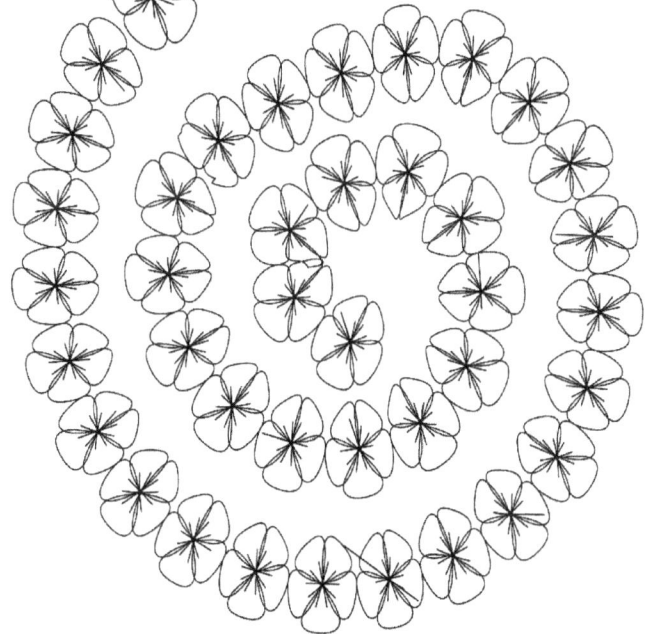

Day / Date : _____

Meal	Details	Calories
Breakfast		
Snack		
Lunch		
Snack		
Dinner		

Exercise	Time	Wt.	Sets/Reps
			/
			/
			/
			/
			/
			/
			/
			/
			/
			/
			/

Today's Results :

Blood Pressure /Time/Pulse :

/   __:__   _____

/   __:__   _____

Today's Weight :

Total Calories :

Water Intake :

Current Medications / Supplements :

What Inspired Me Today? (Ex: A Person, Goal Achieved, A Quote, or Misc.) :

_____

_____

_____

_____

My Progress Notes :

_____

_____

_____

_____

_____

My Progress Reflections
& General Inspirations

_____

_____

_____

_____

_____

_____

_____

_____

_____

_____

_____

_____

_____

_____

_____

_____

Day / Date : _____

Meal	Details	Calories
Breakfast		
Snack		
Lunch		
Snack		
Dinner		

Exercise	Time	Wt.	Sets/Reps
			/
			/
			/
			/
			/
			/
			/
			/
			/
			/
			/

Today's Results :

Blood Pressure /Time/Pulse :

/ ___:___ _____
/ ___:___ _____

Today's Weight :

Total Calories :

Water Intake :

Current Medications / Supplements :

What Inspired Me Today? (Ex: A Person, Goal Achieved, A Quote, or Misc.) :

My Progress Notes :

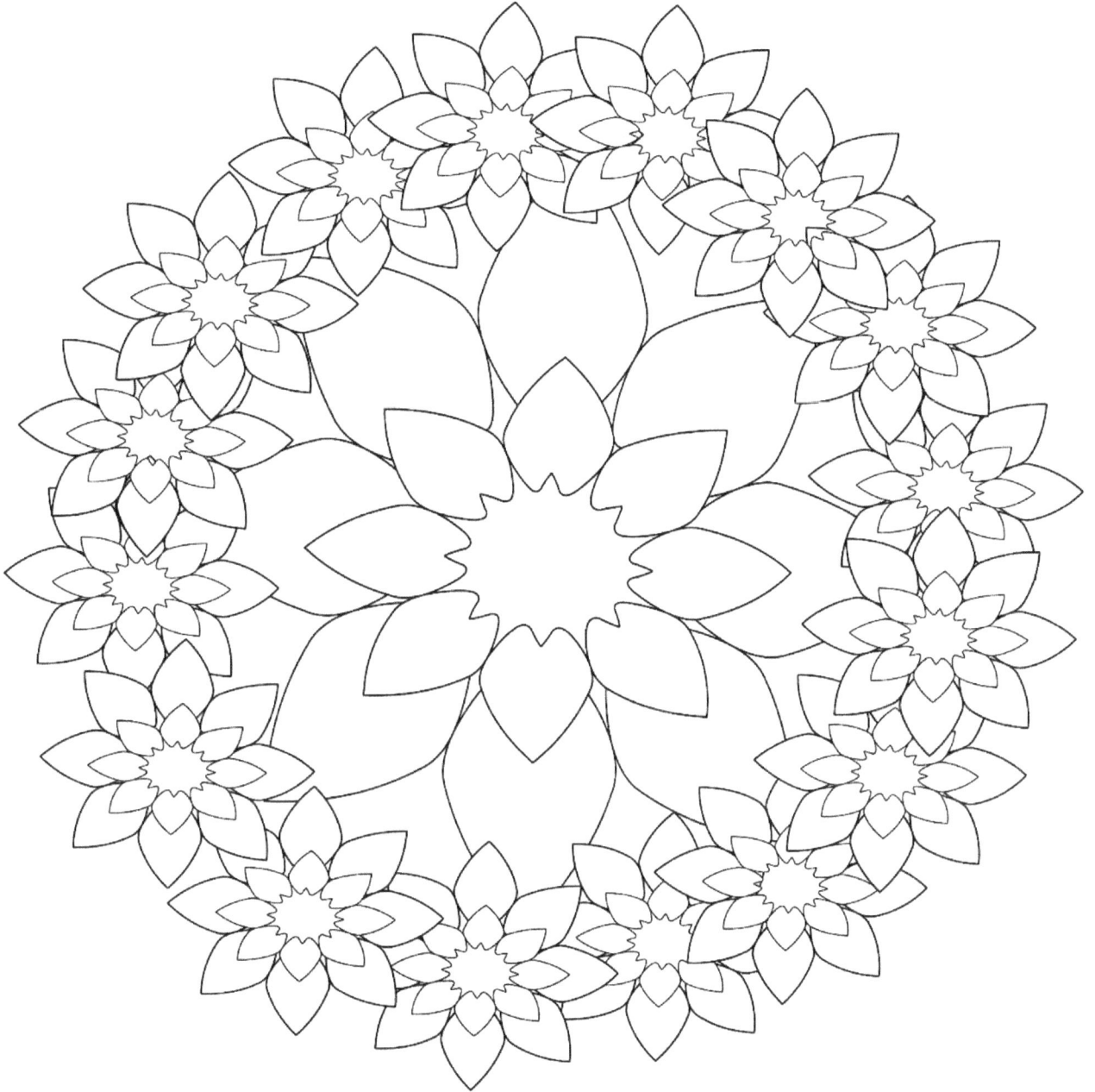

Day / Date : _____

Meal	Details	Calories
Breakfast		
Snack		
Lunch		
Snack		
Dinner		

Exercise	Time	Wt.	Sets/Reps
			/
			/
			/
			/
			/
			/
			/
			/
			/
			/
			/

Today's Results :

Blood Pressure / Time / Pulse :

/   __:__   _____

/   __:__   _____

Today's Weight :

Total Calories :

Water Intake :

Current Medications / Supplements :

What Inspired Me Today? (Ex: A Person, Goal Achieved, A Quote, or Misc.) :

My Progress Notes :

My Progress Reflections
& General Inspirations

_____

_____

_____

_____

_____

_____

_____

_____

_____

_____

_____

_____

_____

_____

_____

_____

Day / Date : _____

Meal	Details	Calories
Breakfast		
Snack		
Lunch		
Snack		
Dinner		

Exercise	Time	Wt.	Sets/Reps
			/
			/
			/
			/
			/
			/
			/
			/
			/
			/
			/
			/

Today's Results :

Blood Pressure /Time/Pulse :

/   __:__   _____

/   __:__   _____

Today's Weight :

Total Calories :

Water Intake :

Current Medications / Supplements :

What Inspired Me Today? (Ex: A Person, Goal Achieved, A Quote, or Misc.) :

My Progress Notes :

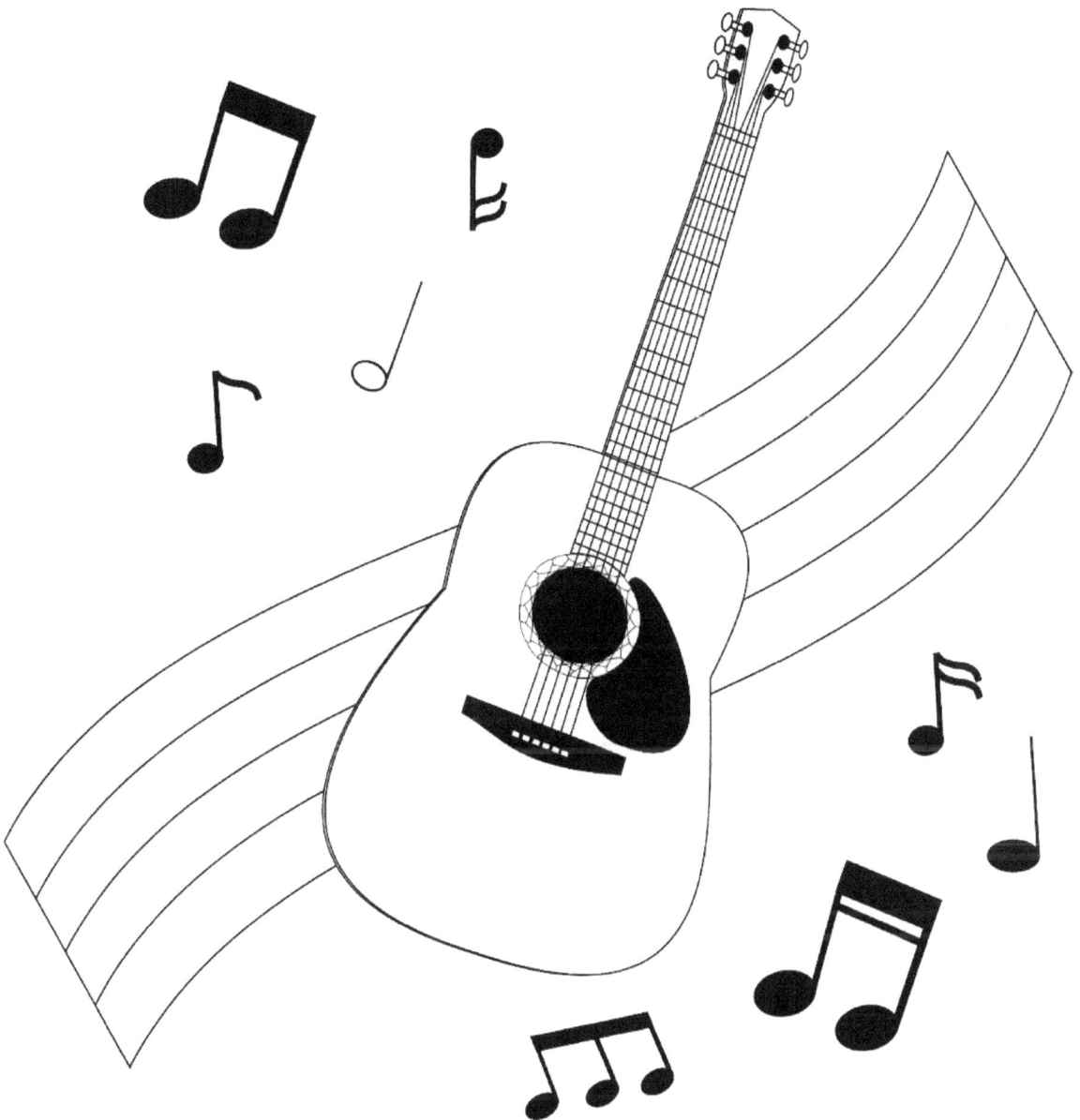

Day / Date : _____

Meal	Details	Calories
Breakfast		
Snack		
Lunch		
Snack		
Dinner		

Exercise	Time	Wt.	Sets/Reps
			/
			/
			/
			/
			/
			/
			/
			/
			/
			/
			/
			/

Today's Results :

Blood Pressure / Time / Pulse :

   /   __:__   _____
   /   __:__   _____

Today's Weight :

Total Calories :

Water Intake :

Current Medications / Supplements :

What Inspired Me Today? (Ex: A Person, Goal Achieved, A Quote, or Misc.) :

My Progress Notes :

My Progress Reflections
& General Inspirations

_____

_____

_____

_____

_____

_____

_____

_____

_____

_____

_____

_____

_____

_____

_____

_____

Day / Date : _____

Meal	Details	Calories
Breakfast		
Snack		
Lunch		
Snack		
Dinner		

Exercise	Time	Wt.	Sets/Reps
			/
			/
			/
			/
			/
			/
			/
			/
			/
			/
			/
			/

Today's Results :

Blood Pressure /Time/Pulse :

/   __:__   _____

/   __:__   _____

Today's Weight :

Total Calories :

Water Intake :

Current Medications / Supplements :

What Inspired Me Today? (Ex: A Person, Goal Achieved, A Quote, or Misc.) :

_____

_____

_____

_____

My Progress Notes :

_____

_____

_____

_____

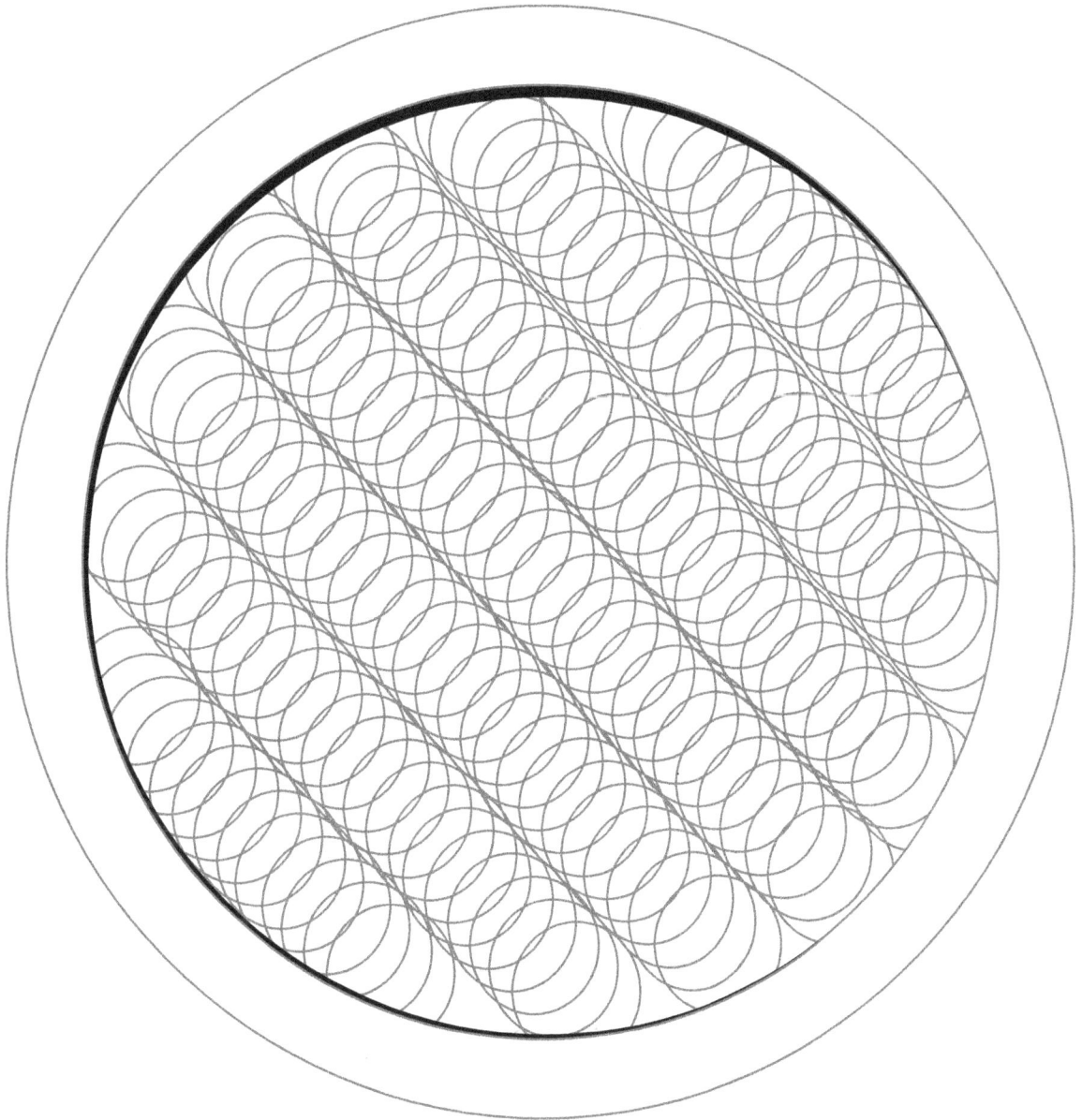

Day / Date : _____

Meal	Details	Calories
Breakfast		
Snack		
Lunch		
Snack		
Dinner		

Exercise	Time	Wt.	Sets/Reps
			/
			/
			/
			/
			/
			/
			/
			/
			/
			/
			/

Today's Results :

Blood Pressure /Time/Pulse :

/   __:__   _____

/   __:__   _____

Today's Weight :

Total Calories :

Water Intake :

Current Medications / Supplements :

What Inspired Me Today? (Ex: A Person, Goal Achieved, A Quote, or Misc.) :

_____

_____

_____

_____

My Progress Notes :

_____

_____

_____

_____

My Progress Reflections
& General Inspirations

_____

_____

_____

_____

_____

_____

_____

_____

_____

_____

_____

_____

_____

_____

_____

_____

_____

Day / Date : _____

Meal	Details	Calories
Breakfast		
Snack		
Lunch		
Snack		
Dinner		

Exercise	Time	Wt.	Sets/Reps
			/
			/
			/
			/
			/
			/
			/
			/
			/
			/
			/
			/

Today's Results :

Blood Pressure /Time/Pulse :
/ __:__ _____
/ __:__ _____

Today's Weight :

Total Calories :

Water Intake :

Current Medications / Supplements :

What Inspired Me Today? (Ex: A Person, Goal Achieved, A Quote, or Misc.) :

My Progress Notes :

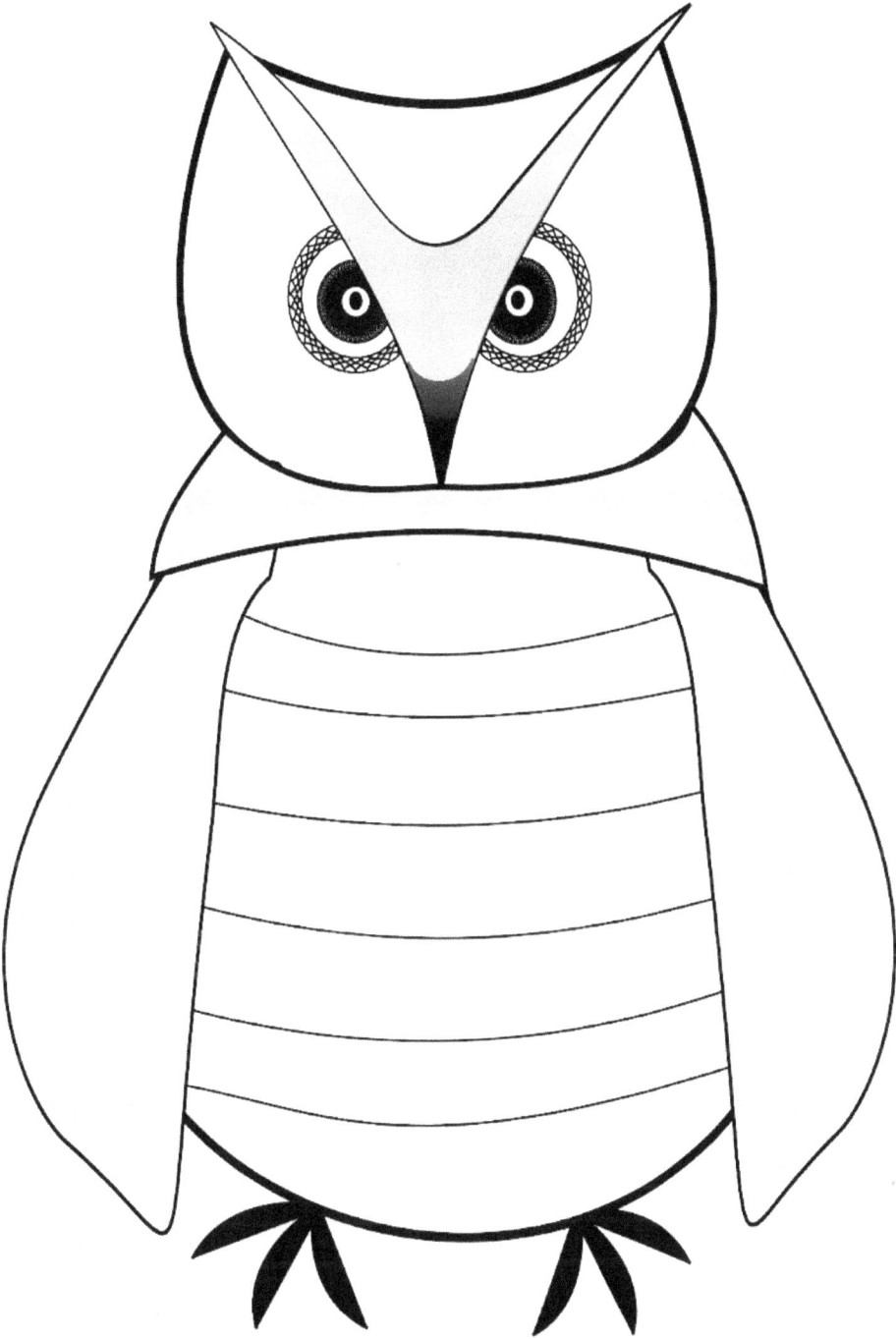

Day / Date : _____

Meal	Details	Calories
Breakfast		
Snack		
Lunch		
Snack		
Dinner		

Exercise	Time	Wt.	Sets/Reps
			/
			/
			/
			/
			/
			/
			/
			/
			/
			/
			/

Today's Results :

Blood Pressure / Time / Pulse :

/ ___:___ _____
/ ___:___ _____

Today's Weight :

Total Calories :

Water Intake :

Current Medications / Supplements :

What Inspired Me Today? (Ex: A Person, Goal Achieved, A Quote, or Misc.) :

My Progress Notes :

My Progress Reflections
& General Inspirations

_____
_____
_____
_____
_____
_____
_____
_____
_____
_____
_____
_____
_____
_____

Day / Date : _____

Meal	Details	Calories
Breakfast		
Snack		
Lunch		
Snack		
Dinner		

Exercise	Time	Wt.	Sets/Reps
			/
			/
			/
			/
			/
			/
			/
			/
			/
			/
			/
			/

Today's Results :

Blood Pressure / Time/Pulse :

/ ___:___ _____

/ ___:___ _____

Today's Weight :

Total Calories :

Water Intake :

Current Medications / Supplements :

What Inspired Me Today? (Ex: A Person, Goal Achieved, A Quote, or Misc.) :

My Progress Notes :

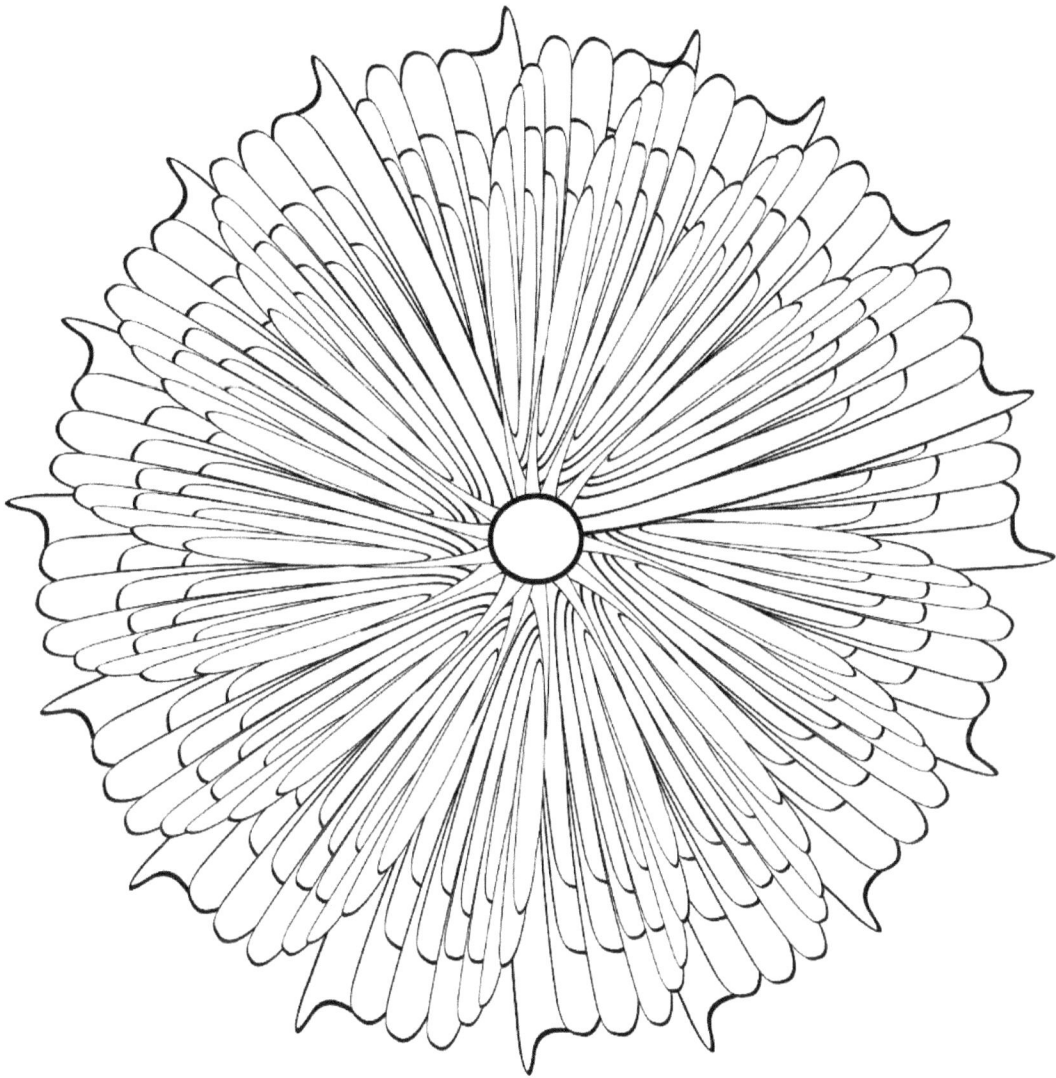

Day / Date : _____

Meal	Details	Calories
Breakfast		
Snack		
Lunch		
Snack		
Dinner		

Exercise	Time	Wt.	Sets/Reps
			/
			/
			/
			/
			/
			/
			/
			/
			/
			/
			/
			/

Today's Results :

Blood Pressure /Time/Pulse :

/ ___:___ _____

/ ___:___ _____

Today's Weight :

Total Calories :

Water Intake :

Current Medications / Supplements :

What Inspired Me Today? (Ex: A Person, Goal Achieved, A Quote, or Misc.) :

My Progress Notes :

My Progress Reflections
& General Inspirations

_____

_____

_____

_____

_____

_____

_____

_____

_____

_____

_____

_____

_____

_____

_____

_____

Day / Date : _____

Meal	Details	Calories
Breakfast		
Snack		
Lunch		
Snack		
Dinner		

Exercise	Time	Wt.	Sets/Reps
			/
			/
			/
			/
			/
			/
			/
			/
			/
			/
			/
			/

Today's Results :

Blood Pressure /Time/Pulse :

/   __:__   _____

/   __:__   _____

Today's Weight :

Total Calories :

Water Intake :

Current Medications / Supplements :

What Inspired Me Today? (Ex: A Person, Goal Achieved, A Quote, or Misc.) :

_____

_____

_____

_____

My Progress Notes :

_____

_____

_____

_____

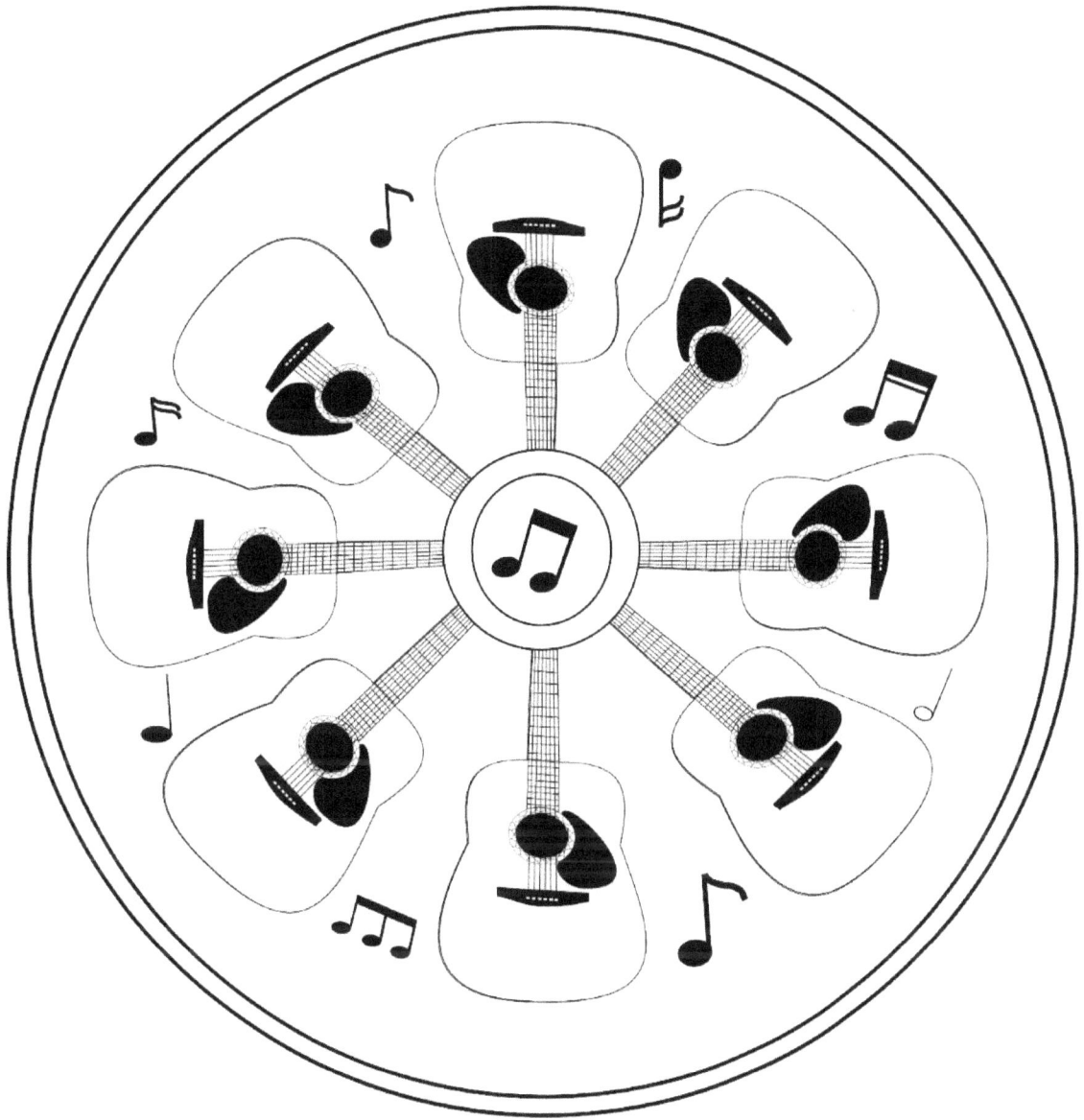

Day / Date : _____

Meal	Details	Calories
Breakfast		
Snack		
Lunch		
Snack		
Dinner		

Exercise	Time	Wt.	Sets/Reps
			/
			/
			/
			/
			/
			/
			/
			/
			/
			/
			/
			/

Today's Results :

Blood Pressure /Time/Pulse :

/ _ _ : _ _ _____

/ _ _ : _ _ _____

Today's Weight :

Total Calories :

Water Intake :

Current Medications / Supplements :

What Inspired Me Today? (Ex: A Person, Goal Achieved, A Quote, or Misc.) :

My Progress Notes :

My Progress Reflections
& General Inspirations

_____

_____

_____

_____

_____

_____

_____

_____

_____

_____

_____

_____

_____

_____

_____

_____

_____

Day / Date : _____

Meal	Details	Calories
Breakfast		
Snack		
Lunch		
Snack		
Dinner		

Exercise	Time	Wt.	Sets/Reps
			/
			/
			/
			/
			/
			/
			/
			/
			/
			/
			/

Today's Results :

Blood Pressure /Time/Pulse :

/ __:__ _____

/ __:__ _____

Today's Weight :

Total Calories :

Water Intake :

Current Medications / Supplements :

What Inspired Me Today? (Ex: A Person, Goal Achieved, A Quote, or Misc.) :

_____

_____

_____

_____

My Progress Notes :

_____

_____

_____

_____

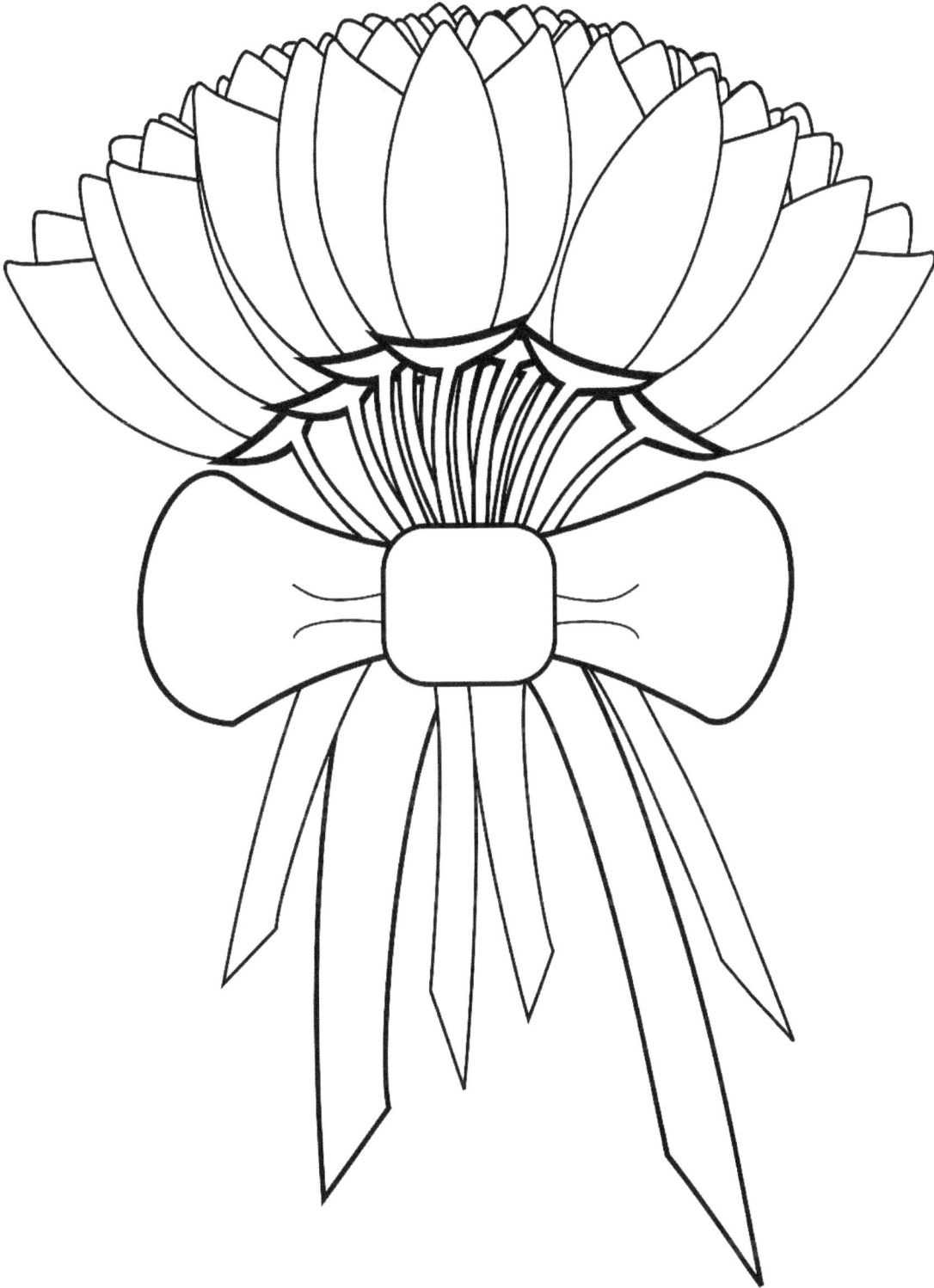

Day / Date : _____

Meal	Details	Calories
Breakfast		
Snack		
Lunch		
Snack		
Dinner		

Exercise	Time	Wt.	Sets/Reps
			/
			/
			/
			/
			/
			/
			/
			/
			/
			/
			/
			/

Today's Results :

Blood Pressure /Time/Pulse :

/ ___:___ _____

/ ___:___ _____

Today's Weight :

Total Calories :

Water Intake :

Current Medications / Supplements :

What Inspired Me Today? (Ex: A Person, Goal Achieved, A Quote, or Misc.) :

My Progress Notes :

My Progress Reflections
& General Inspirations

_____

_____

_____

_____

_____

_____

_____

_____

_____

_____

_____

_____

_____

_____

_____

_____

Day / Date : _____

Meal	Details	Calories
Breakfast		
Snack		
Lunch		
Snack		
Dinner		

Exercise	Time	Wt.	Sets/Reps
			/
			/
			/
			/
			/
			/
			/
			/
			/
			/
			/

Today's Results :

Blood Pressure /Time/Pulse :

/ ___:___ _____

/ ___:___ _____

Today's Weight :

Total Calories :

Water Intake :

Current Medications / Supplements :

What Inspired Me Today? (Ex: A Person, Goal Achieved, A Quote, or Misc.) :

_____

_____

_____

_____

My Progress Notes :

_____

_____

_____

_____

_____

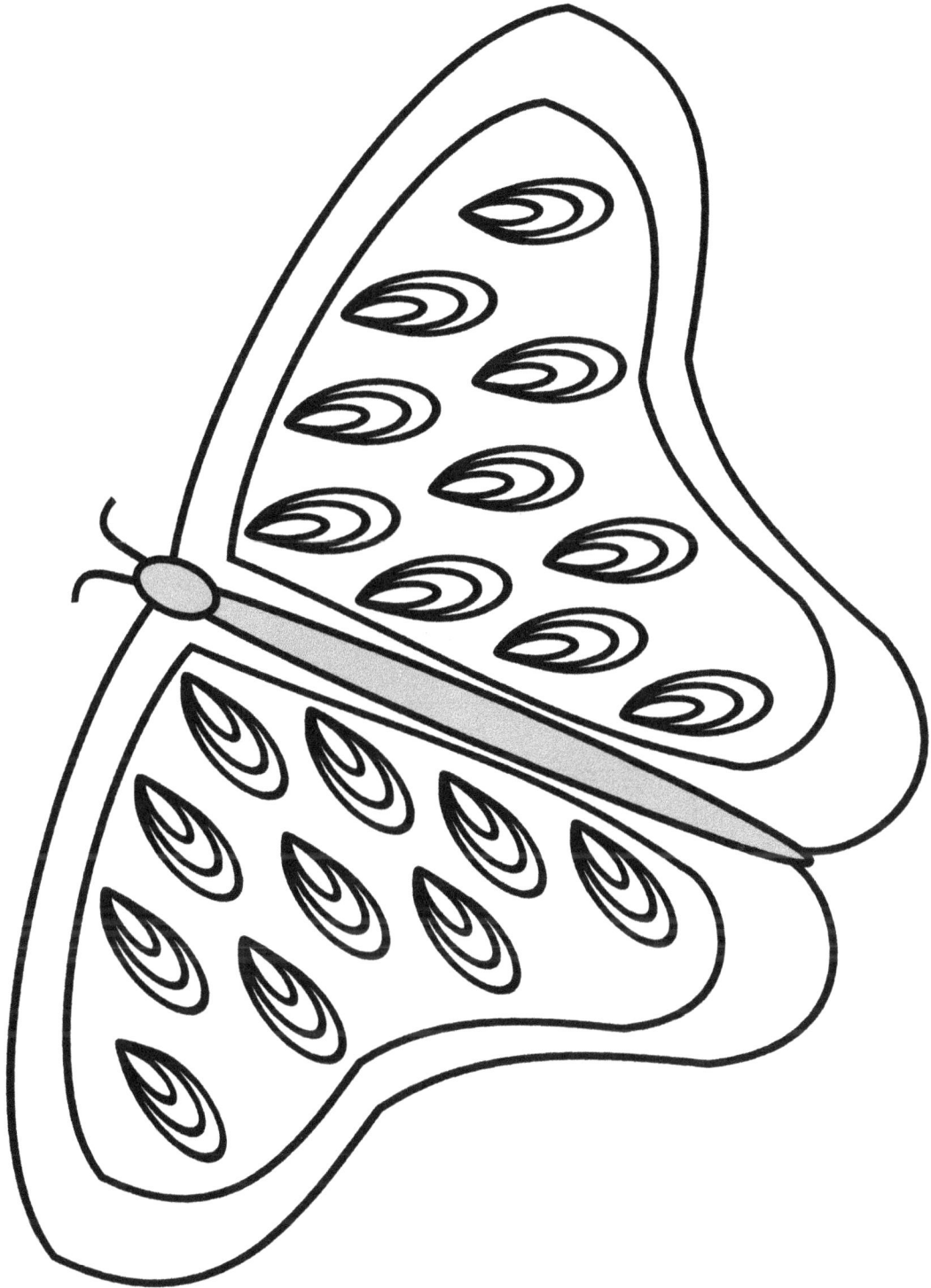

Day / Date : _____

Meal	Details	Calories
Breakfast		
Snack		
Lunch		
Snack		
Dinner		

Exercise	Time	Wt.	Sets/Reps
			/
			/
			/
			/
			/
			/
			/
			/
			/
			/
			/

Today's Results :

Blood Pressure /Time/Pulse :

/ _____ __:__ _____

/ _____ __:__ _____

Today's Weight :

Total Calories :

Water Intake :

Current Medications / Supplements :

What Inspired Me Today? (Ex: A Person, Goal Achieved, A Quote, or Misc.) :

My Progress Notes :

My Progress Reflections
& General Inspirations

_____

_____

_____

_____

_____

_____

_____

_____

_____

_____

_____

_____

_____

_____

_____

_____

_____

Other Titles by This Author

The Friendship Oyster

Getting Ready for School: My Morning Routine
Written with Michael Keen (age 10)
Illustrated by Rosita Henley

Our Day at Universal: A Visit to Two Parks In One Day
A Brothers' Review
Written with Jessie Keen (age 12) & Michael Keen (age 10)

Anticipated Titles

JAX and Allie: Beach Fun
Illustrated by Melissa Keen

Our New Orleans Visit
A Brothers' Review
Written with Jessie Keen (age 13) & Michael Keen (age 10)

JAX and Allie: Going to the Mardi Gras

How I Wrote and Illustrated My First Book

Follow us on Facebook for anticipated release dates
and for additional titles
Contact: sandra@keeninspirationalmedia.com

THANK YOU FOR READING AND FOR
SUPPORTING WHAT WE DO.

WE LOVE WHAT WE DO!

www.ingramcontent.com/pod-product-compliance
Lightning Source LLC
Chambersburg PA
CBHW080050280326
41934CB00014B/3271